The Progressive Nature of Renal Disease: Myths and Facts

Contributions to Nephrology

Vol. 75

KARGER

Basel · München · Paris · London · New York · New Delhi · Singapore · Tokyo · Sydney

2nd Verona Seminar on Nephrology, September 29–October 1, 1988

The Progressive Nature of Renal Disease: Myths and Facts

Editors
Lamberto Oldrizzi, Giuseppe Maschio, Carlo Rugiu, Verona;
Vito M. Campese, Los Angeles, Calif.

39 figures and 34 tables, 1989

KARGER

Basel · München · Paris · London · New York · New Delhi · Singapore · Tokyo · Sydney

Contributions to Nephrology

Library of Congress Cataloging-in-Publication Data
Verona Seminar on Nephrology (2nd : 1988)
The progressive nature of renal disease: myths and facts / 2nd Verona Seminar on Nephrology, September 29–October 1, 1988; editors, Lamberto Oldrizzi ... [et al.].
p. cm.–(Contributions to nephrology; vol. 75)
Includes bibliographical references.
1. Kidneys–Diseases–Congresses. I. Oldrizzi, Lamberto, 1954–. II. Title. III. Series.
[DNLM: 1. Kidney Diseases–Congresses. W1 C0778UN v. 75/WJ 300 V548p]
RC902.A2V47 1988 616.6′1–dc20 DNLM/DLC
ISBN 3-8055-5021-9

Bibliographic Indices
This publication is listed in bibliographic services, including Current Contents® and Index Medicus.

Drug Dosage

The authors and the publisher have exerted every effort to ensure that drug selection and dosage set forth in this text are in accord with current recommendations and practice at the time of publication. However, in view of ongoing research, changes in government regulations and the constant flow of information relating to drug therapy and drug reactions, the reader is urged to check the package insert for each drug for any change in indications and dosage and for added warnings and precautions. This is particularly important when the recommended agent is a new and/or infrequently employed drug.

Printed in Switzerland by Thür AG Offsetdruck, Pratteln
ISBN 3-8055-5021-9

Contents

Counteracting Progression in Clinical Practice

Nutritional Problems in the Uremic Patient

Preface

The Second Verona Seminar on Nephrology was entirely devoted to the mechanisms of progression of chronic renal disease. The four main sessions included reports from leading scientists from the USA, Sweden, France, Federal Republic of Germany, England and Italy.

The first session explores the mechanisms of progression in experimental renal disease. The roles of immunologic factors, prostaglandins, platelets, disordered mineral metabolism, hypertension, gut hormones, and dietary components are discussed. In addition, the potential role of reduced renal mass, either congenital or acquired, is presented as an important modulator of the renal susceptibility to either hypertension or renal failure.

The second session examines progression in human renal disease. The natural history of glomerulonephritidis, tubulointerstitial nephropathy, reflux nephropathy, inherited renal disease, hypertensive vascular nephropathy, and diabetic nephropathy is presented with regard to the mechanism of progression.

The third session is devoted to the possibility of counteracting progression in clinical practice. Dietary and nondietary intervention is discussed, with particular emphasis on new antihypertensive agents.

The fourth session examines the nutritional problems in the uremic patient. Some metabolic abnormalities typically observed in the uremic state, the amino acid imbalance and the optimal protein intake in patients with chronic renal failure are reviewed, as well as the modalities to assess the nutritional status in these patients.

The meeting was attended by an audience of over 350 persons and the scientific level was considered to be excellent.

We hope that the reader will find these proceedings both enjoyable and useful for future studies on a rather hot topic in nephrology.

Once again, we express our deep gratitude to Merck Sharp & Dohme, Italy, and to Ciba Geigy, Italy, for the generous financial support to the publication of these proceedings.

Giuseppe Maschio,
Vito M. Campese,
Lamberto Oldrizzi,
Carlo Rugiu

Oldrizzi L, Maschio G, Rugiu C, et al. (eds): The Progressive Nature of Renal Disease: Myths and Facts. Contrib Nephrol. Basel, Karger, 1989, vol 75, pp 1–12

Immunopathology and Progression of Experimental Renal Disease[1]

G. Camussi[a, b], *C. Tetta*[b], *G. Montrucchio*[b], *E. Turello*[b], *A. Vercellone*[b]

[a]Cattedra di Nefrologia Sperimentale, Dipartimento di Biochimica e Biofisica, I Facoltà di Medicina e Chirurgia, Università di Napoli, Napoli; [b]Laboratorio di Immunopatologia, Istituto di Nefro-Urologia, Cattedra di Nefrologia, Università di Torino, Torino, Italia

A complex array of factors contribute to the expression and progression of immune glomerular injury: (1) the nature of the initiating mechanism namely the antibody, or the immune complex or a T-cell-mediated mechanism; (2) the intensity and the persistence of the initiating mechanism; (3) the recruitment and local action of inflammatory cells; (4) the response of intrinsic glomerular cells.

The final event in progressive glomerular diseases is scar formation leading to obliteration of the glomerular filter (glomerulosclerosis) and eventually chronic renal failure. The final effector that determines glomerulosclerosis is the local cellular response to injury.

While the pathogenetic mechanism initiating glomerular injury is disease-specific, the cellular response to injury is rather monomorphic. Its expression is an altered proliferation of resident glomerular cells and matrix production. As in other vascularized tissues, glomerular injury usually results in an inflammatory response that may initiate the process of repair and healing or the scar formation leading to glomerulosclerosis.

In glomeruli, the acute, transient, inflammatory response determines hyperplasia of endothelial, mesangial and visceral epithelial cells and/or changes in glomerular basement membrane (GBM) and mesangial matrix. These alterations may be reversed when the initiating mechanism disappears and chronic renal failure does not occur, as seen in experimentally induced acute serum sickness or sometimes in human post-infectious glomerulonephritis.

An incongruous or sustained activation of the mechanisms involved in the inflammatory response may result not in protection but rather in tissue

[1] Part of the studies reported in this publication were supported by grants from Ministero 40% Ricerca Nazionale, 'Progressione dell'Insufficienza Renale, Genesi e Prevenzione', progetto, 'Mediatori della Flogosi Glomerulare'.

injury, thus ensuing in irreversible functional impairment. Glomerular inflammation may progress to irreversible sclerosis and loss of function as result of: (1) massive acute glomerular injury such as that seen in necrotizing vasculitis, Goodpasture's glomerulonephritis or in experimental nephrotoxic nephritis; (2) a sustained disease process due to persistence of the initiating mechanism or of the biologic sequelae triggered by such a mechanism.

Recently researchers have focused on the factors that may determine an altered growth of resident glomerular cells and production of extracellular matrix as these are the hallmarks of progressive glomerular disease. From these studies two possibilities have emerged: (1) the persistence of the initiating pathogenetic mechanism that influences the behaviour of glomerular cells directly or indirectly through the release of inflammatory mediators; (2) an altered 'regulation' of the behaviour of glomerular cells triggered by the initiating inflammatory stimulus which persists despite the disappearance of the pathogenetic stimulus.

The initiating insult may determine an increased expression of genes coding for the synthesis of peptide growth factors or of matrix components that maintain an altered proliferative and secretory response of resident glomerular cells.

Progression of Glomerular Injury in Experimental Models of Immune Glomerular Pathology

Immune deposits in glomeruli may be formed by antibodies reacting with structural glomerular antigens such as components of the GBM, or antigens expressed on the plasma membranes of intrinsic glomerular cells (in situ formed immune complexes) or by deposition of circulating antigen-antibody complexes [for review see ref. 1, 2]. The concomitant activation of cells of the delayed hypersensitivity response may contribute to the expression of glomerular injury. Besides its nature, the intensity and duration of the initiating stimulus as well as its localization in the glomerular structures may condition the clinico-morphological expression of glomerular immune injury.

In nephrotoxic nephritis, the first, acute, inflammatory response triggered by the interaction of heterologous antibodies reacting with GBM antigens is sustained by the late 'autologous' phase due to binding of the host's antibodies to the planted heterologous immunoglobulins [3]. The expression of the disease is dependent on the activation of complement [4] and the recruitment of inflammatory cells (polymorphonuclear neutrophils, PMN, monocytes/macrophages and platelets) [5, 6]. The massive insult of glomeruli that is associated with fibrinoid necrosis is followed by the progressive impairment of renal function [3]. Tissue necrosis as well as release by inflammatory or resident glomerular cells of cytokines influencing the growth of resident glomerular cells and matrix production may contribute to the evolution to glomerular sclerosis. It has been reported that besides the increased production of antigens normally present in the mesangium, such as type IV collagen, fibronectin and laminin, types I, III and V collagen is also present in sclerotic glomeruli during anti-GBM antibody disease in the rat [7]. It is unclear whether the presence of interstitial collagen within the glomeruli depends only on rupture of Bowman's capsule followed by ingrowth of fibroblasts from the periglomerular interstitium or from mesangial cells that have been shown to be able to produce also type III collagen in culture [8, 9]. Since interstitial collagen may promote mesangial cell proliferation in vitro, it is conceivable that also in vivo newly expressed matrix constituents may contribute to modulating the proliferative behaviour of resident glomerular cells [8, 10–12].

The site of formation of immune deposits may also be relevant to the expression of glomerular injury. Fries et al. [13] have shown that a single implantation of immune complexes in the subendothelial-mesangial space determines a transient inflammatory response with their rapid removal and healing in the absence of cell proliferation. On the other hand, a transient proliferative response was observed in experimentally induced acute serum sickness [14] and in the Vogt's model of acute exudative glomerulonephritis [15] due to implantation of a cationized antigen in the glomerular capillary wall of preimmunized rats where deposits are formed both in the subendothelium and in the subepithelium. In these models the accumulation of inflammatory cells is associated with proliferation of resident glomerular cells that, however, regresses with the regression of inflammation. In these models, the initiating stimuli persist only for a limited period of time and so do inflammatory lesions and proliferation of resident glomerular cells which occur only in the presence of the immunologic stimuli.

Heymann nephritis may be considered a chronic disease of the kidney in which significant immunologic injury occurs only during the limited period in which antibodies are present in the circulation. Functional deficits of the glomeruli and tubules measured late in the natural course of Heymann nephritis may reflect the permanent and irreparable damage produced during the immunologically active phase of the disease. Reimmunization with FxlA late in the course of Heymann nephritis is followed by severe alterations in morphology and function of both glomeruli and tubules [16]. Thus, repeated immunologic insults may also be a cause of progression of glomerular disease.

Recently, van Lew et al. [17] have attempted to establish a relationship between kidney function to immunopathology in chronic serum sickness of rats. The initiating stimulus in this model, i.e. the chronic immunization with bovine serum albumin (BSA), is persistent even if the nature of the stimulus varies with time in relation to the individual immunologic response. Three categories (mild, moderate and severe) of kidney disease were identified from the analysis of kidney function in rats with chronic serum sickness and corresponded to distinct stages of kidney immunopathology. In rats with mild disease immune deposits were limited to the mesangium; proliferation and accumulation of inflammatory cells were slight or absent. In rats with moderate disease despite maintainance of normal total kidney glomerular filtration rate, a moderate decrease of single nephron glomerular filtration rate was observed. Urinary protein excretion and plasma composition were characteristic of the nephrotic syndrome. The immune deposits were present along the glomerular capillary wall as well as in the mesangium and were associated with proliferation and accumulation of inflammatory cells. In rats with severe chronic serum sickness, the decrease of total kidney glomerular filtration rate and of single nephron glomerular filtration rate were associated with a diffuse proliferative glomerulonephritis. Significant proteinuria persisted. However, the very low glomerular filtration rate limited the total glomerular loss of protein. Immune deposits primarily present in the glomerular capillary wall were not significantly increased in respect of the moderate stage of the disease. However, diffuse proliferation and infiltration of inflammatory cells and segmental fibrinoid necrosis were observed in glomeruli. Precipitating antibodies to BSA were no longer detectable in the circulation and the discontinuation of antigen administration was not associated with the recovery of kidney function. In this model, therefore, the disease may eventually progress independently from the initiating stimulus.

Preliminary results in our laboratory indicate that mesangial cells cultured from rat kidney in the severe stage of the disease produce an increased amount of interleukin (IL-1), even in the absence of the initiating stimulus.

These results may suggest that the primary insult might change the secretory phenotype of glomerular cells inducing or increasing the expression of genes coding for polypeptide growth factors and matrix constituents. The end result is therefore a disregulation of growth and biosynthetic behaviour of intrinsic glomerular cells. In agreement with this hypothesis are the results of Werber et al. [18] showing an augmented expression of the gene coding for IL-1 by glomerular mesangial cells of rats with immune complex glomerulonephritis. A novel and enhanced IL-1 gene expression was also described in mice with lupus nephritis [19]. Ebihara et al. [20] recently described an enhanced expression of mRNA for glycoproteins such as units of type IV collagen and B_1 chain of laminin in a murine model of polycystic kidney disease.

The technology derived from molecular biology promises to give us in the future more information about the capacity and regulation of glomerular cells to synthesize matrix components, cytokines, enzymes and other mediators in normal and pathological conditions.

Polypeptide Mediator Network

The 'polypeptide mediator network' defines the network of interacting signals that regulate growth, differentiation and function of cells involved in immunity, inflammation and haematopoiesis [21]. The list of polypeptide mediators that includes interleukins (IL-1, 2, 3, 4), γ-interferons (IFN), tumor necrosis factor (TNF), granulocyte colony-stimulating factor (G-CSF), monocyte colony-stimulating factor (M-CSF) and so on has grown rapidly during the past decade. Several of these factors may be produced locally in the kidney by recruited inflammatory and T cells and/or by resident glomerular cells.

Inflammatory Cells

Several findings suggest the involvement of macrophages in glomerular immune injury [6, 22–24]. Macrophages may produce IL-1, TNF and G-CSF [20]. TNF by itself is also a signal for macrophages to produce IL-1, autacoids and platelet-activating factor (PAF) that are all mediators capable of amplifying the inflammatory reaction and local cell proliferation [21, 25, 26]. In addition, IL-1 activates T cells directly or through accessory cells [27] and activated T cells produce IL-2, a T cell growth factor, G-CSF, IL-3, a haematopoietic growth factor, IL-4, a B cell growth factor and IFN [21]. IFN activates in turn macrophages and amplifies TNF production by macrophages [26, 27]. In addition, TNF increases major histocompatibility complex antigens in endothelial cells, alters their growth and morphological pattern, increases the synthesis of procoagulant activity and enhances endothelial cell adhesiveness for inflammatory cells [26]. Both IL-1 and TNF stimulate synthesis and release of PAF [28, 29].

Expression of tissue factor and of activation antigens was demonstrated in the endothelia of glomeruli exposed to IL-1, endotoxin (LPS) or TNF in vitro [30, 31]. IFN [32] and TNF [26] induce expression of class II antigens by cultured endothelial cells and TNF promotes morphologic rearrangement of these cells facilitating trans-endothelial trafficking [26]. In addition, antibodies directed against antigens expressed by human cultured endothelial cells exposed to LPS, IL-1 or TNF are present in sera from patients with Kawasaki vasculitis [33, 34]. It has been recognized that intrinsic glomerular cells express class II antigens in normal conditions or after exposure to cytokines [23, 35–37]. Ia or Ia-like molecules are required for antigen presentation and development of T-cell-mediated hypersensitivity [38]. Ia-positive macrophages are present in the rat mesangium and respond to mitogenic challenge in a genetically restricted fashion [36, 37].

The expression of class II molecules by glomerular endothelial cells activated by monokines endows these cells with an important role in presenting antigens to sensitized T cells. Although a small number of T lymphocytes are present in glomeruli of rats with nephrotoxic glomerulonephritis [39–41], and T lymphocytes in glomeruli of patients with proliferative glomerulonephritis are quite variable in number [42, 43], it is not yet firmly established whether T cells infiltrate glomeruli and whether they may influence accumulation of phagocytic monocytes [42, 43].

After implantation of subnephritogenic amounts of rabbit anti-GBM antibodies or immune complexes containing rabbit IgG in the glomeruli of rats, proliferation of glomerular cells and infiltration of macrophages occur only when rats receive T cells from donors sensitized to rabbit IgG [44, 45]. These experiments suggest a role for cytokines derived from T lymphocytes in inducing glomerular injury. An additional evidence for the role of T cells in glomerular pathology derives from the study of B-cell-deficient chickens immunized with GBM that develop proliferative, crescentic glomerulonephritis without immune deposits [46]. In addition, the disease may be transferred by infusing sensitized T lymphocytes to syngeneic chickens [47].

Increasing evidence suggests that an important factor in the progression of glomerulonephritis is the interstitial infiltration of T cells and Ia-positive monocyte-macrophages that has been found in various forms of glomerulonephritis recognizing different initiating mechanisms [48, 49].

The involvement of platelets in glomerular pathology is relevant not only for the release of mediators that may influence glomerular permeability and the recruitment of inflammatory cells, but also for the potential role of platelet cationic proteins in inducing proliferation of resident glomerular cells and production of matrix [50]. The low-affinity platelet factor 4 (PF4), and the basic protein platelet-derived growth factor (PDGF) are all mitogenic for fibroblasts and PDGF exerts the same action on smooth muscle cells [50]. PDGF in addition has a growth-promoting effect on many types of mesenchymal cells including glomerular endothelial and mesangial cells [51, 52].

Even if the role of PDGF in determining glomerular hypercellularity in vivo remains to be proven, a few experimental data correlate the intraglomerular platelet activation with mesangial cell proliferation [53] and with focal glomerular sclerosis [54]. The local production of these mediators may orchestrate in the kidney inflammatory and proliferative events and may influence matrix production (fig. 1).

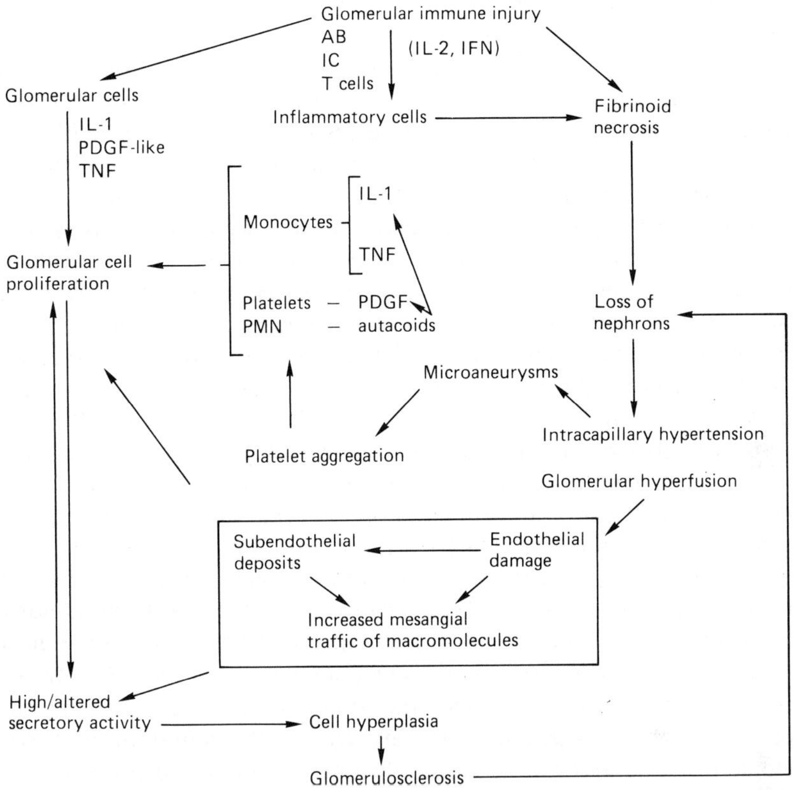

Fig. 1. Progression of glomerular immune injury: role of inflammatory mediators. AB = Antibody; IC = immune complexes.

Resident Glomerular Cells

In addition to inflammatory cells, resident glomerular cells may contribute to the production of several factors that are part of the 'polypetide mediator network' [reviewed in ref. 55]. Mesangial cells, provided that they are actively proliferating, produce IL-1 [56]. While non-cycling mesangial cells do not express IL-1 mRNA, cycling mesangial cells express IL-1 mRNA resulting in synthesis and release of IL-1 [57]. IL-1 mRNA expression in synchronized cells may be induced by a defined combination of peptide growth factors such as PDGF, EGF, insulin, and transferrin [57]. Human mesangial cells in culture express also the genes for the A and B chains (c-sis) of PDGF and may produce and release PDGF [58, 59]. Preliminary results in our laboratory indicate that LPS-stimulated mesangial cells release TNF and other cytokines that might affect the behaviour of resident glomerular and inflammatory cells. In fact it has been recently reported that TNF stimulates the release of PDGF from cultured endothelial cells [60]. The observation that glomerular cells in culture are able to produce growth promoting factors and matrix glycoproteins suggests an autocrine self-regulation of their replicative and secretory activities [56].

In fact IL-1 and PDGF have been shown to promote proliferation of mesangial and endothelial cells [51, 52, 61]. The induction of plasma membrane-associated protein kinase activity by IL-1 seems to be the mechanism whereby IL-1 initiates mesangial cell activation [62]. PDGF also increases collagen synthesis and may alter the phenotypic pattern of collagen secretion [63]. The production of matrix from glomerular cells appears of critical importance for the progression of glomerular injury. Since PDGF as well as G-CSF preferentially bind to several matrix constituents, the composition of matrix may influence cell growth [64, 65]. IL-1 may also affect matrix turnover either by stimulating collagen type IV synthesis and secretion of neutral metalloendopeptidases which degrade denaturated types I, III and native IV collagen [66]. In addition, matrix itself may modulate the behaviour of glomerular cells [67]. Fibronectin and collagen, for instance, may facilitate attachment and growth of mesangial cells [12], while polyanionic heparin exerts an inhibitory effect [68, 69]. Since heparan sulphate proteoglycans are normal constituents of GBM [70] and mesangium [71], they may have a negative control on mesangial cell proliferation. It may be envisaged that persistent autocrine stimulation of growth and matrix production by glomerular cells may trigger the initial proliferation of glomerular cells and the altered production of matrix that contribute to the progression of glomerular disease (fig. 1).

In conclusion, the progression of glomerular disease may be sustained by an acute massive glomerular injury or by a persistent immunologic stimulus inducing both an altered regulation of growth of resident glomerular cells and of matrix production. However, glomerular injury may progress also after the disappearance of the initiating pathogenetic stimulus as a result of loss of self-regulation of replicative and secretory activities of glomerular cells.

References

1 Hoedemaker J: Experimental glomerulonephritis; in Davison, Nephrology. London, Baillière, 1988, vol I, pp 409–440.

2 Andres G, Brentjens JR, Caldwell PRB, et al: Biology of disease. Formation of immune deposits and disease. Lab Invest 1986;55:510–520.

3 Unanue ER, Dixon FJ: Experimental glomerulonephritis, immunological events and pathogenetic mechanisms. Adv Immunol 1967;6:1–90.

4 Unanue ER, Dixon FJ: Experimental glomerulonephritis. IV. Participation of complement in nephrotoxic nephritis. J Exp Med 1964;122:99–116.
5 Cochrane CG, Unanue ER, Dixon FJ: A role of polymorphonuclear leukocytes and complement in nephrotoxic nephritis. J Exp Med 1965;122:99–116.
6 Holdsworth SR, Neale TJ, Wilan CB: Abrogation of macrophage-dependent injury in experimental glomerulonephritis in the rabbit. Use of anti-macrophage serum. J Clin Invest 1981;68:686–698.
7 Foellmer HG, Sterzel RB, Kashgarian M: Progressive glomerular sclerosis in experimental antiglomerular basement membrane glomerulonephritis. Am J Kidney Dis 1986;VII:5–11.
8 Striker GE, Striker LJ: Biology of disease: Glomerular cell culture. Lab Invest 1985;53:122–131.
9 Adler S, Striker LJ, Striker GE, et al: Studies of progressive glomerular sclerosis in the rat. J Pathol 1986;123:553–562.
10 Harper PA, Robinson JM, Hoover RL, et al: Improved methods for culturing rat glomerular cells. Kidney Int 1984;26:875–880.
11 Oberley TD, Murphy PJ, Steinert BW, et al: A morphologic and immunofluorescent analysis of primary guinea pig glomerular cell types grown in chemically defined media: evidence for clonal growth and cell differentiation. Virchows Arch [Cell Pathol] 1982;41:145–170.
12 Dunn MJ, Michaels S: Fibronectin and adhesive glycoproteins stimulate proliferation of quiescent mesangial cells (Abstract). Kidney Int 1988;33:154.
13 Fries JWU, Mendrick DL, Rennke HG: Determinants of immune complex-mediated glomerular injury. Kidney Int 1988;34:333–345.
14 Dixon FJ: The pathogenesis of glomerulonephritis. Am J Med 1968;44:493–498.
15 Vogt A, Rohrbach R, Shimizu F: Interaction of cationized antigen with rat glomerular basement membrane: in situ immune complex formation. Kidney Int 1982;22:27–35.
16 Noble B, Van Liew JB, Brentjens JR, et al: Effect of reimmunization with FxlA late in the course of Heymann nephritis. Lab Invest 1982;47:427–436.
17 Van Liew JB, Brentjens JR, Noble B: Relationship of kidney function to immunopathology in chronic serum sickness of rats. Kidney Int 1983;24:160–169.
18 Werber HI, Emancipator SN, Tykocinski ML, et al: The interleukin-1 gene is expressed by rat glomerular mesangial cells and is augmented in immune complex glomerulonephritis. J Immunol 1987;138:3207–3212.
19 Boswell J, Yui M, Burt D, et al: Novel and enhanced interleukin 1 gene expression in lupus nephritis (Abstract). Kidney Int 1988;33:150.
20 Ebihara I, Killen PD, Laurie GW, et al: Altered messanger RNA expression of basement membrane components in a murine model of polycystic kidney disease. Lab Invest 1988;58:262–269.
21 Old LJ: Polypeptide mediator network. Nature 1987;326:330.
22 Atkins RC, Holdsworth SR, Glasgow EF, et al: The macrophage in human rapidly progressive glomerulonephritis. Lancet 1976;i:830–832.
23 Unanue ER, Schreiner GF, Cotran RS: A role of mononuclear phagocytes in immunologically induced glomerulonephritis; in Cummings NB, Michael AF, Wilson CB (eds): Immune Mechanisms in Renal Disease. New York, Plenum Press, 1983, pp 443–453.
24 Schreiner GF, Cotran RS, Pardo V, et al: A mononuclear cell component in experimental immunological glomerulonephritis. J Exp Med 1978;147:369–384.
25 Shalaby MR, Pennica D, Palladino M: An overview of the history and biological properties of tumor necrosis factor. Springer Semin Immunopathol 1986;9:33–49.

26 Beutler B, Cerami A: Cachectin: more than a tumor necrosis factor. N Engl J Med 1987;316:379–385.
27 Dinarello CA: Interleukin-1 and the pathogenesis of the acute phase response. N Engl J Med 1984;411:1413–1418.
28 Camussi G, Bussolino F, Salvidio G, et al: Tumor necrosis factor/Cachectin stimulates rat peritoneal macrophages, polymorphonuclear neutrophils and human endothelial cells to synthesize and release platele-activating factor. J Exp Med 1987;166:1390–1404.
29 Bussolino F, Camussi G, Baglioni C: Synthesis and release of platelet-activating factor by human vascular endothelial cells treated with tumor necrosis factor or Interleukin-1. J Biol Chem, in press.
30 Bevilacqua MP, Pober JS, Wheeler ME, et al: Interleukin-1 activation of vascular endothelium. Effects on procoagulant activity and leukocyte adhesion. Am J Pathol 1985;121:394–403.
31 Bevilacqua MP, Pober JS, Majeau GR, et al: Recombinant tumor necrosis factor induces procoagulant activity in cultured human vascular endothelium: characterization and comparison with the actions of Interleukin-1. Proc Natl Acad Sci USA 1986;83:4533–4537.
32 Pober JS, Gimbrone MA, Cotran RS, et al: Ia expression by vascular endothelium is inducible by activated T cells and by human gamma-interferon. J Exp Med 1983;157:1339–1353.
33 Leung DYM, Collins T, Lapierre LA, et al: IgM antibodies present in the acute phase of Kawasaki syndrome lyse cultured vascular endothelial cells stimulated by gamma interferon. J Clin Invest 1986;77:1428–1435.
34 Leung DYM, Geha RS, Newberge JW, et al: Two monokines, Interleukin-1 and tumor necrosis factor, render cultured vascular endothelial cells susceptible to lysis by antibodies circulating during Kawasaki syndrome. J Exp Med 1986;164:1958–1972.
35 Mayrhofer G, Schon-Hegrad MA: Ia antigens in rat kidney, with special reference to their expression in tubular epithelium. J Exp Med 1983;157:2097–2109.
36 Schreiner GF, Cotran RS, Pardo V, et al: A mononuclear cell component in experimental immunological glomerulonephritis. J Exp Med 1978;147:369–384.
37 Schreiner GF, Kiely JM, Cotran RS, et al: Characterization of resident glomerular cells in the rat expressing Ia determinants and manifesting genetically restricted interactions with lymphocytes. J Clin Invest 1981;68:920–931.
38 Unanue ER, Allen PM: Comment on the finding of Ia expression in nonlymphoid cells (Editorial). Lab Invest 1986;55:123–125.
39 Tipping PG, Neale TJ, Holdsworth SR: T lymphocyte participation in antibody-induced experimental glomerulonephritis. Kidney Int 1985;27:530–537.
40 Boyce NW, Tipping PG, Holdsworth SR: Lymphokine (MIF) production by glomerular T lymphocytes in experimental glomerulonephritis. Kidney Int 1986;30:673–677.
41 Eldredge C, Wiggins RC: T cells in the glomerulus, periglomerular region and around venules early in crescentic nephritis in the rabbit. Evidence for glomerulo-interstitial signals (Abstract). Kidney Int 1987;31:318.
42 Nolasco FEB, Cameron JS, Hartley B, et al: Intraglomerular T cells and monocytes in nephritis: study with monoclonal antibodies. Kidney Int 1987;31:1160–1166.
43 Hooke DH, Gee DC, Atkins RC: Leukocyte analysis using monoclonal antibodies in human glomerulonephritis. Kidney Int 1987;31:964–972.
44 Bhan AK, Schneeberger EE, Collins AB, et al: Evidence for a pathogenic role of cell-mediated immune mechanism in experimental glomerulonephritis. J Exp Med 1978;148:246–260.

45 Bhan AK, Collins AB, Schneeberger EE, et al: A cell mediated reaction against glomerular-bound immune complexes. J Exp Med 1979;150:1410–1420.
46 Bolton WK, Tucker FL, Sturgill C: New avian model of experimental glomerulonephritis consistent with mediation by cellular immunity. J Clin Invest 1984;73:1263–1276.
47 Chandra M, Tyson T, Sturgill B, et al: Transfer of experimental autoimmune glomerulonephritis in chicken by sensitized cells (Abstract). Kidney Int 1985;27:208.
48 Boucher A, Droz D, Adafer E, et al: Characterization of mononuclear cell subsets in renal cellular interstitial infiltrates. Kidney Int 1986;29:1043–1049.
49 Brunati C, Brando B, Confalonieri R, et al: Immunophenotyping of mononuclear cell infiltrates associated with renal disease. Clin Nephrol 1986;26:15–20.
50 Barnes JL, Venkatachalam MA: The role of platelets and polycation mediators in glomerular vascular injury. Semin Nephrol 1985;5:57–68.
51 Striker GE, Killen PD, Farin FM: Human glomerular cell in vitro isolation and characterization. Transplant Proc 1980;22:88–98.
52 Striker GE, Soderland C, Bowen-Pope DF, et al: Isolation, characterization and propagation in vitro of human glomerular endothelial cells. J Exp Med 1984;160:323–328.
53 Cattel V: Focal mesangial proliferative glomerulonephritis in the rat caused by Habu snake venom: The role of platelets. Br J Exp Pathol 1979;60:201–208.
54 Torgensen L, Glynn MF, Horig T, et al: Renal lesions and rise in blood pressure caused by adenosyne diphosphate-induced platelet aggregation in rabbits. Lab Invest 1970;23:347–357.
55 Lovett DH, Sterzel RB: Cell culture approaches to the analysis of glomerular inflammation. Kidney Int 1986;30:246–254.
56 Lovett DH, Szamel M, Ryan JL, et al: Interleukin-1 and the glomerular mesangium. I. Purification and characterization of a mesangial cell-derived autogrowth factor. J Immunol 1986;136:3700–3705.
57 Lovett DH, Larsen A: Cell cycle-dependent expression of IL-1 messenger-RNA in human mesangial cells (Abstract). Kidney Int 1987;31:325.
58 Abboud HE, Poptic E, DiCorleto P: Production of by rat mesangial cells in culture. J Clin Invest 1987;80:675–683.
59 Abboud HE, Silver B, DiCorleto P, et al: Human mesangial cells in culture express the genes for the A and B chain (S.C-SIS) of platelet-derived growth factor (PDGF): regulation by thrombin (Abstract). Kidney Int 1988;33:148.
60 Hajjar K, Hajjar DP, Silverstein RL, et al: Tumor necrosis factor-mediated release of platelet-derived growth factor from cultured endothelial cells. J Exp Med 1987;166:235–245.
61 Lovett DH, Ryan JL, Sterzel RB: Stimulation of rat mesangial cell proliferation by macrophage interleukin-1. J Immunol 1983;131:2830–2836.
62 Lovett D, Martin M, Bursten S, et al: Interleukin-1 and the glomerular mesangium III. IL-1-dependent stimulation of mesangial cell protein kinase activity. Kidney Int 1988;34:26–35.
63 Ross PM, Raines EW, Bowenpop DF: The biology of platelet-derived growth factor. Cell 1986;46:155–169.
64 Smith J, Singh J, Lillquist J, et al: Growth factors adherent to cell substrate are mitogenically active in situ. Nature 1982;296:154–156.
65 Gordon MY, Riley GP, Watt SM, et al: Compartmentalization of haematopoietic growth factor (GM-CSF) by glycosaminoglycans in the bone marrow microenvironment. Nature 1987;326:403–405.

66 Martin J, Lovett DH, Gemsa D, et al: Enhancement of glomerular mesangial cell neutral proteinase secretion by macrophages: role of Interleukin-1. J Immunol 1986 ;137:525–529.

67 Gospodarowicz D, Delgado D, Vlodavsky I: Permissive effect of the extracellular matrix on cell proliferation in vitro. Proc Natl Acad Sci USA 1980;77:4094–4098.

68 Castellot JJ, Hoover RL, Harper PA, et al: Heparin and glomerular epithelial cell-secreted heparin-like species inhibit mesangial cell proliferation. Am J Pathol 1986;125:493–500.

69 Castellot JJ, Hoover RL, Harnovsky MJ: Glomerular endothelial cells secrete a heparin-like inhibitor and a peptide stimulator of mesangial cell proliferation. Am J Pathol 1985;120:427–435.

70 Stow JL, MacKay K, Striker LJ, et al: Basement membrane heparan sulfate proteoglycans (BMHSPG) synthesized by cultured glomerular epithelial cells (GEC) (Abstract). Kidney Int 1988;33:174.

71 Van der Woude FJ, Brown DM, Kim YK, et al: Characterization of de novo proteoglycans (PG) synthesized by cultured human glomerular visceral epithelial cells (GEVC) and mesangial cells (MES) (Abstract). Fed Proc 1987;46:1230.

Giovanni Camussi, MD Laboratorio di Immunopatologia,
Istituto di Nefro-Urologia, Cattedra di Nefrologia,
Università di Torino, I–10126 Torino (Italy)

Oldrizzi L, Maschio G, Rugiu C, et al. (eds): The Progressive Nature of Renal Disease: Myths and Facts. Contrib Nephrol. Basel, Karger, 1989, vol 75, pp 13–18

Role of Prostaglandins in Experimental Renal Disease

Thomas H. Hostetter, Karl A. Nath

Division of Renal Diseases, University of Minnesota, Minneapolis, Minn., USA

Renal prostaglandin production exerts a controlling influence on renal function during physiologic and pathophysiologic stresses. A large number of experimental chronic renal diseases provide evidence for the roles of various prostaglandin species in determining renal function [1, 2]. Moreover, it has been well recognized that in clinical chronic renal diseases of various types, inhibition of prostaglandin synthesis can exert deleterious effects on renal hemodynamics, as well as variable effects on protein excretion, potassium balance, and water metabolism. Prostaglandins appear to have varying influences in various models. A well-established simple model of chronic renal insufficiency is the subtotal nephrectomy model achieved by unilateral nephrectomy and partial ablation of the residual kidney. The rat subjected to this procedure develops, first, compensatory growth and functional changes in residual nephrons followed by arterial hypertension, proteinuria, increasing glomerular sclerosis, and progressive uremia [3]. The view has arisen that the early compensatory changes exert injurious effects leading to the late adverse consequences [4]. This review will focus on the role of prostaglandins in the early compensation and late injury in this model.

Compensatory Hypertrophy

With reduction in renal mass, the residual nephrons undergo dramatic adaptation. They enlarge, a process conventionally termed compensatory hypertrophy, signifying the greater increase in cell mass than cell number. The signal or signals which initiate this compensatory renal growth are poorly understood; however, evidence exists for the possibility that local renal production of prostaglandins might contribute to this adaptive renal growth. In vitro studies with myocytes and renal tubular cells have demonstrated effects of prostaglandins in stimulating cell growth [3, 5]. In the case of the rabbit renal proximal tubular cells, the studies have documented an increase in cell size with addition of PGE_1 in micromolar concentrations to culture media [6]. Although this level of PGE_1 may exceed that found in vivo, these studies in conjunction with others employing nonrenal cells, do suggest the possibility that the prostaglandins can directly stimulate or at least, in concert with other elements, sustain renal compensatory growth.

Perhaps the most direct evidence for a role of prostaglandins in compensatory renal growth derives from experiments of Logan et al. [7]. In these studies, rats underwent simple unilateral nephrectomy, and were given either indomethacin at 5.0 mg/kg/day or vehicle. Two days following uninephrectomy, the residual kidney in vehicle treated animals had grown by 32 mg in dry weight, whereas the residual kidney of animals treated during the 2 days following nephrectomy with indomethacin, increased by only 9 mg. In addition, the intrarenal levels of PGE_2 and 6 keto $PGF_{1\alpha}$ were augmented in the residual kidneys of animals administered vehicle, and these augmentations were obliterated by indomethacin treatment. Finally, these studies demonstrated that indomethacin also limited the compensatory increases in protein and RNA content of the residual kidneys.

Compensatory Hemodynamic Changes

A wide array of nephron functions becomes altered with compensatory renal growth [8]. However, the striking and perhaps critical alterations are increases in renal blood flow and GFR to residual nephrons. These hemodynamic alterations, in a sense, set the agenda for associated alterations in sodium reabsorption, potassium excretion, and acid elimination.

Even before alterations in the renal blood flows are established after partial renal ablation, increases in renal lymphatic flows and peritubular interstitial pressure have been described [9]. These changes in interstitial dynamics likely reflect changes in vasomotor control of the renal microcirculation, particularly the peritubular capillary circulation. However, the exact hemodynamic genesis of the observed early changes in lymphatic behavior has not been described in detail. Nevertheless, these shifts in intrarenal fluid dynamics do depend on local prostaglandin synthesis. Evidence for this assertion derives from studies of Hahne and Persson [9]. In their studies, lymphatic flow, sodium excretion, and urine flow increased from the remaining kidney in the first hour following contralateral nephrectomy. In association, there was a 50% increase in subcapsular hydrostatic pressure, an index of interstitial pressure. With inhibition of prostaglandin synthesis prior to nephrectomy, augmentation of lymphatic flow, diuresis, and natriuresis were blunted following contralateral nephrectomy. The authors concluded that prostaglandin synthesis was critical to these early functional changes, and they further speculated that these changes in interstitial dynamics were integral to the pursuant changes in blood flow and filtration rate, perhaps via the tubulo-glomerular feedback system [9, 10].

Inhibition of prostaglandin synthesis in the setting of chronic renal disease reduces renal blood flow and glomerular filtration rate (GFR) as demonstrated by clinical studies. Kirschenbaum and Serros [11] have reported a similar effect in the rabbit with subtotal nephrectomy. To determine the more precise hemodynamic mechanism, whereby the chronically reduced GFR depends on prostaglandin synthesis, Nath et al. [12] examined the subtotal nephrectomy model in the rat. The studies, conducted 3–5 weeks following subtotal nephrectomy (a time at which compensatory increases in renal mass, as well as renal hemodynamic function, are fully established). Indomethacin was administrated acutely to determine the degree to which the hemodynamic adaptations depended upon local prostaglandin production. Intravenous indomethacin led to significant reductions in whole kidney and superficial single nephron GFR due to falls in renal blood flow, and the glomerular ultrafiltration coefficient. But these changes were observed only in the animals with subtotal nephrectomy, not in control animals having two kidneys with a full complement of nephrons. The reduction in single nephron GFR with prostaglandin synthesis inhibition, equalled approximately half of the compensatory increment in single nephron GFR in the baseline state. In other words, at least half of the compensatory elevation of single nephron GFR, could be attributed to local prostaglandin production. Since, in separate studies, this dose of indomethacin reduced urinary excretion of prostaglandins by only about 50%, prostaglandin production appears to account for at least half, and perhaps more, of the sustained elevation in single nephron filtration rate.

Studies by Stahl et al. [13] reported that in vitro glomeruli obtained from rats having undergone subtotal nephrectomy produced greater amounts of prostaglandin products than glomeruli from normal rats, and these differences obtained when the augmented production rates were expressed per milligram of glomerular protein or per glomerulus. In accord with these findings, Nath et al. [12] reported increased urinary excretion rates per nephron for PGE, 6-keto-$PGF_{1\alpha}$, and thromboxane ($TBXA_2$) in rats with subtotal nephrectomy compared to control rats with two kidneys. These and other studies support the view that increased prostaglandin production and excretion occurs in the residual nephron, and that these products subserve the increase in blood flow and GFR.

Injurious Role of Prostaglandins

The general view has arisen that the compensatory alterations of the remnant nephron, particularly the hemodynamic ones, may serve to maintain homeostasis and mitigate the falls of whole kidney function over the short term, but over the longer term, adversely affect the structure and function of these nephrons [4]. Furthermore, to the degree that augmented prostaglandin production sustains compensatory changes, at least certain of these autacoids would be responsible for the chronic injury. Two general approaches have been applied in attempts to discern the role of prostaglandin synthesis in progressive renal injury in the remnant kidney model, dietary lipid manipulation and prostaglandin synthesis inhibition.

Barcelli et al. [14] fed a diet supplemented with linoleic acid to rats subjected to subtotal nephrectomy. The rationale for this dietary manipulation was that linoleic acid can serve as precursor to arachidonic acid. Thus, supplementation of linoleic in the diet, should increase rather nonspecifically prostaglandin production. These studies demonstrated that the progressive rise in serum creatinine sustained by animals on a diet not supplemented by linoleate was significantly blunted by linoleic acid supplementation. Also, proteinuria and histologic evidence of sclerotic glomeruli were diminished in the animals fed the high linoleic diet. The effects of the diet on renal prostaglandin production are somewhat more difficult to interpret. The rates of prostaglandin production were measured in renal slices in vitro. The high linoleic diet augmented PGE production in the cortex, but had no effect on thromboxane synthesis. In addition, there was no greater rate of prostaglandin production per milligram protein in partially nephrectomized animals, regardless of diet. Since the protein content per nephron rises with compensatory growth, an increased PGE production per residual nephron, and per glomerulus as shown by others, likely obtained even in these slices from animals with reduced renal mass. A similar beneficial result of dietary linoleic acid supplementation on renal function have been reported by Heifets et al. [15]. However, in this latter series of investigations, the salutary effects of linoleic acid supplementation were associated with significantly lower arterial pressures, an effect not observed by Barcelli et al. [14]. While the precise physiologic and biochemical mechanisms underlying the protective effect of linoleic acid supplementation require more investigation, these studies clearly emphasize that this supplementation, in particular, and alteration of renal prostaglandin production, in general, can influence renal damage.

Thromboxane synthesis blockade has been employed to investigate the role of this product on renal injury in the ablation model. Purkerson et al. [16] administered a thromboxane synthesis inhibitor (OKY 158) to rats with subtotal nephrectomy. Thromboxane excretion was augmented in the subtotal nephrectomized rat compared to control rats with two kidneys, but this augmentation was blocked by the inhibitor. Furthermore, renal dysfunction was also diminished after 5 weeks of administration of the drug. Specifically, proteinuria was substantially less, and the GFR was higher in the animals maintained on the blocking agent. In addition, arterial pressure was reduced in rats maintained on this drug. The authors emphasized the effects of the agent on inhibiting platelet aggregation, and suggested its beneficial effects were due to a reduction in intraglomerular platelet thrombosis. Another interpretation, and one which does not exclude an effect on platelets, is that by lowering the arterial pressure, hemodynamically mediated injury was diminished.

Eicosapentaenoic acid (EPA) can serve as a substrate for cyclooxygenase. The triene products are analogous to the diene series derived from arachidonate as a substrate. However, they have different biological potency. In particular, the $TBXA_3$ derived from EPA, is relatively inert compared to $TBXA_2$, while PGI_3 has the same range of potency as PGI_2 derived from arachidonate. These observations have lead to a large number of studies employing dietary supplementation of EPA, usually from fish oil. Murine lupus nephritis responds favorably to dietary supplementation with EPA [17]. However, recent studies by Scharschmidt et al. [18] demonstrated an adverse effect of such supplementation (compared to a beef tallow supplemented diet) on the remnant kidney model. EPA supplementation led to significantly greater serum creatinine, greater proteinuria, and lower GFR in the supplemented animals. In addition, renal histological evaluation confirmed that there was a greater percentage of sclerosed glomeruli in animals ingesting the fish oil enriched diet. Of incidental interest, the serum levels of cholesterol and triglycerides, which are typically elevated in animals with subtotal nephrectomy, were diminished to near normal by fish oil supplementation. This incidental finding indicates that normalization of plasma lipids is not sufficient to mitigate the renal injury in this model since the animals with the normalization of plasma lipid levels had the worse injury. The investigators attributed the deleterious effects of EPA supplementation to a resultant greater inhibition of vasodilator prostaglandins relative to vasoconstrictive $TBXA_2$. Thus, they speculate that their ratios were adversely affected in favor of $TBXA_2$. Although the physiologic and cellular mechanisms, whereby, such an imbalance would generate glomerular sclerosis is uncertain, this speculation again suggests an especially injurious role for $TBXA_2$.

References

1 Patrono C, Dunn MJ: The clinical significance of inhibition of renal prostaglandin synthesis. Kidney Int 1987;32:1–12.

2 Rahman MA, Stork JE, Dunn MJ: The roles of eicosanoids in experimental glomerulonephritis. Kidney Int 1987;32:S40–S48.

3 Shimamura T, Morrison AB: A progressive glomerulosclerosis occurring in partial five-sixths nephrectomized rats. Am J Pathol 1975;79:95–106.

4 Brenner BM, Meyer TW, Hostetter TH: Dietary protein intake and the progressive nature of kidney disease: the role of hemodynamically mediated glomerular injury in the pathogenesis of progressive glomerular sclerosis in aging, renal ablation and intrinsic renal disease. N Engl J Med 1982;307:652–657.

5 Palmer RM, Reeds PJ, Atkinson T, Smith RH: The influence of changes in tension on protein synthesis and prostaglandin release in isolated rabbit muscles. Biochem J 1983;214:1011–1014.

6 Fine LG, Badie-Dezfooly B, Lowe AG, Hamzeh A, Wells J, Salehmoghaddam S: Stimulation of Na^+/H^+ antiport is an early event in hypertrophy of renal proximal tubular cells. Proc Natl Acad Sci USA. 1985;82:1736–1740.

7 Logan JL, Lee SM, Benson B, Michael UF: Inhibition of compensatory renal growth by indomethacin. Prostaglandins 1986;31:253–261.

8 Hayslett JP: Functional adaptation to reduction in renal mass. Physiol Rev 1979;59:137–164.

9 Hahne B, Persson AEG: Prevention of interstitial pressure change at unilateral nephrectomy by prostaglandin synthesis inhibition. Kidney Int 1984;25:42–46.

10 Hahne B, Selen G, Persson AEG: Indomethacin inhibits renal functional adaptation to nephron loss. Renal Physiol 1984;7:13–21.

11 Kirschenbaum MA, Serros ER: Effect of prostaglandin inhibition on glomerular filtration rate in normal and uremic rabbits. Prostaglandins 1981;22:245–254.

12 Nath KA, Chmielewski DH, Hostetter TH: Regulatory role of prostanoids in glomerular microcirculation of remnant nephrons. Am J Physiol 1987;252:F829–F837.

13 Stahl RA, Kudelka S, Paravicini M, Schollmeyer P: Prostaglandin and thromboxane formation in glomeruli from rats with reduced renal mass. Nephron 1986;42:252–257.

14 Barcelli U, Weiss M, Pollak VE: Effects of a dietary prostaglandin precursor on the progression of experimentally induced chronic renal failure. J Lab Clin Med 1982;100:786–797.

15 Heifets M, Morrissey JJ, Purkerson ML, Morrison AR, Klahr S: Effect of dietary lipids on renal function in rats with subtotal nephrectomy. Kidney Int 1987;32:335–341.

16 Purkerson ML, Joist JH, Yates J, Valdes A, Morrison A, Klahr S: Inhibition of thromboxane synthesis ameliorates the progressive kidney disease of rats with subtotal renal ablation. Proc Natl Acad Sci USA 1985;82:193–197.

17 Prickett JD, Robinson DR, Steinberg AD: Dietary enrichment with the polyunsaturated fatty acid eicosapentaenoic acid prevents proteinuria and prolongs survival in NZB × NZWf1 mice. J Clin Invest 1981;68:556–559.

18 Scharschmidt LA, Gibbons NB, McGarry L, et al: Effects of dietary fish oil on renal insufficiency in rats with subtotal nephrectomy. Kidney Int 1987;32:700–709.

Dr. Thomas H. Hostetter, Department of Medicine, Renal Division,
University of Minnesota, 516 Delaware St. SE, Minneapolis, MN 55455 (USA)

Oldrizzi L, Maschio G, Rugiu C, et al. (eds): The Progressive Nature of Renal Disease: Myths and Facts. Contrib Nephrol. Basel, Karger, 1989, vol 75, pp 19–25

Acute Renal Effects of Protein and Amino Acids: The Potential Role of Gastrointestinal Hormones

Anders Alvestrand, Jonas Bergström

Department of Renal Medicine, Karolinska Institute, Huddinge Hospital, Stockholm, Sweden

A diet rich in protein causes a sustained, marked increase in renal blood flow (RBF) and glomerular filtration rate (GFR) in dogs [1–3]. Both acute and chronic effects of dietary protein on renal hemodynamics have also been observed in humans. Thus, several investigators have found that RBF and GFR increase within 30–90 min following the ingestion of a protein-rich meal [4–6]. The acute increases in RBF and GFR following a protein-rich test meal have been observed to be of approximately equal magnitude irrespective of if the subjects have been on a high- or low-protein diet during the preceding days [5–7].

Although the association between protein intake and renal function has been known for many years, the mechanism by which ingested protein enhances GFR has not been established. Renewed interest in the hemodynamic response to dietary protein was aroused by the hypothesis that glomerular hyperfiltration may be harmful by inducing progressive glomerulosclerosis, and that protein-induced increments in GFR contribute to the progressive decline in renal function in chronic renal failure [8]. This hypothesis is mainly based on experiments in rats with subtotal renal ablation, in which protein restriction reduced GFR in the remaining nephrons, prevented further nephron destruction and prolonged survival.

The observations that intravenous infusion of individual amino acids in dogs [9, 10] or mixtures of amino acids in humans [11, 12] augments RBF and GFR suggest that the increase in plasma amino acid concentrations in some way may induce the renal response. However, it is not likely that amino acids have a direct effect on the kidney, since in the isolated perfused kidney supply of amino acids have little [13] or no effect on GFR [14].

Hormonal Stimulation of Renal Hemodynamics after a Protein-Rich Meal or Amino Acid Infusion

It has been suggested that the increase in GFR and RBF after a protein load or amino acid infusion may be mediated by some hormone [8]. The possible role of a hormonal mediator is supported by the observations that the amino acid-induced rise in GFR and RBF is blocked by somatostatin [12, 15]. Studies in humans indicate that somatostatin has no direct effect on the kidney, suggesting that the inhibitory action of somatostatin on renal hemodynamics is related to its ability to inhibit the secretion of some hormone(s) [12]. Somatostatin suppresses secretion of growth hormone, insulin and pancreatic glucagon, and also secretion of all known gut peptides [16].

It is not likely that the renal response to a protein load or an amino acid infusion is mediated by growth hormone, since the changes renal hemodynamics after a protein meal or infusion of arginine in growth hormone-deficient individuals are similar to those observed in healthy subjects [17, 18].

From a teleological point of view it seems logical that GFR increases following a protein meal, and it is attractive to speculate whether some gastrointestinal hormone not only plays a role in the digestive and metabolic processes but also signal the kidney to increase the elimination of nitrogenous waste products.

Although infusion of secretin has been shown to induce increases in RBF and diuresis in humans, it would appear that these effects of secretin are pharmacological effects only [19]. Of the gastrointestinal hormones only glucagon has been shown to have effects on renal hemodynamics when infused in physiological doses.

Effects of Glucagon on Renal Hemodynamics

Glucagon is secreted by the endocrine pancreas after a protein ingestion or intravenous infusion of individual amino acids [20] or amino acid mixtures [5, 12], and glucagon infusion increases RBF and GFR in dogs by dilating renal afferent arterioles [21, 22]. Exogenous infusion of this hormone also enhances GFR in healthy human subjects [23]. Consequently, glucagon has been suggested as a likely mediator of the stimulative effect of protein on renal hemodynamics [8]. Several studies have shown a temporal relationship between the glucagon and GFR peaks after a protein meal [5, 24] or amino acid infusion [12]. Also, a significant correlation between the absolute peak rise in glucagon and GFR has been observed in healthy subjects following infusion of amino acids [12]. It has recently been demonstrated that infusion of the branched-chain amino acids has no stimulative effect on GFR and RBF [25]. Since glucagon secretion is not stimulated by the branched-chain amino acids [24], these results indirectly support the possible role of glucagon as a mediator of the renal response to amino acids.

However, it is not likely that glucagon directly stimulates renal hemodynamics. Studies by Premen et al. [26] demonstrated that intravenous infusion of glucagon at a dose that increases plasma glucagon to a level somewhat higher than that measured following a meat meal failed to alter RBF or GFR from their baseline values. To mimic the postprandial increases in renal hemodynamics, an arterial plasma glucagon level over ten times higher than the peak postprandial level was required.

The Potential Role of a Liver-Derived Factor as Mediator of the Renal Response to Protein

On the basis of experimental and clinical evidence we have recently proposed that glomerular hyperfiltration, after high protein intake, during amino acid infusion, and during glucagon infusion, is caused by increased secretion of such a liver-produced hormone, a common triggering factor being an increase uptake of free amino acids in the liver [27]. This liver-derived factor may exert its stimulative effect on RBF and GFR by selectively reducing the tone of the afferent arterioles.

This hypothesis was based largely on the studies of Uranga and co-workers [28–30], who previously have shown that the liver vein blood from toads, rabbits, and dogs contains a factor, termed glomerulopressin, that enhances GFR in rats and dogs, but does not influence systemic blood pressure. This hormone has been characterized as a glucoronide with a molecular weight of less 500 daltons, which exerts its effect on GFR by dilating the afferent arteriole. Glomerulopressin also increases contractile tension in smooth muscle strips. Inhibition of these effects by indomethacin suggests that they are mediated by prostaglandins. A similar mechanism may be inferred for the effect of glomerulopressin on the glomerulus, but no data have been presented showing this to be the case.

In studies by Uranga et al. [30] intrarenal infusion of a high dose of glucagon failed to increase RBF or GFR, whereas marked elevation of RBF and GFR were observed during infusion of the same dose of glucagon through the portal vein. Glucagon infused into the portal vein also stimulated glomerulopressin production. However, the dose of glucagon infused probably resulted in unphysiologically high portal vein glucagon levels. However, during portal infusion of glucagon at a dose that was calculated to result in a portal vein glucagon concentration lower than that measured following meat ingestion Premen [31] observed elevations in RBF and GFR to approximately the level previously observed in dogs after a meat meal. In contrast there were no changes in renal hemodynamics during intrarenal infusion of the same dose of glucagon. These results, thus, confirm the physiologic importance of the liver during glucagon-induced increases in renal hemodynamics. The mechanism by which the liver mediates the effect of glucagon on RBF and GFR is, however, not clear.

We have speculated that enhanced uptake of free amino acids by the liver, due to increased circulating amino acid concentrations and/or hyperglucagonemia, is a primary stimulus for glomerulopressin secretion [27]. This suggestion accords with results of previous studies which may suggest that increases in GFR after protein or amino acid administration are related to metabolism of amino acids within the liver. Amino acids which are poorly metabolized within the liver do not appear to stimulate renal hemodynamics [9, 25].

In severe liver failure the synthetic functions of the liver are deranged and production of albumin and other liver-derived proteins are decreased. Conceivably, other metabolic functions of the liver are also impaired. If the increases in RBF and GFR after a protein meal or during glucagon infusion depend on a liver-derived hormone, it therefore seems reasonable to anticipate that the effects of such stimuli on renal hemodynamics are blunted in hepatic failure. Dratwa et al. [32] studied the acute effect of protein on GFR in 7 patients with severe liver disease but with normal baseline GFR as determined by creatinine clearances. Measurement of GFR over 2 h after ingestion of 80 g protein showed no change compared with baseline values in the cirrhotics, whereas GFR increased by 24% in a group of healthy control subjects. Another group of patients with advanced cirrhosis studied by Hirschberg et al. [33] showed no increase in GFR after a protein challenge. In dogs with experimental cirrhosis with ascites glucagon infusion did not increase GFR, unlike the effect of glucagon in normal dogs, dogs with renal hypoperfusion, and dogs with chronic partial vena caval obstruction and ascites [34]. These results support the suggestion that the stimulative effect of protein and glucagon on renal hemodynamics is mediated via the liver, and suggest that the sick liver fails to respond appropriately to stimuli that enhance the secretion of a factor with stimulating effects on the kidney. However, the observations of Woods et al. [11], that amino acid infusion stimulates renal hemodynamics in dogs in the absence of a functional liver, contradict the importance of a liver-derived factor as a mediator of the renal response to protein or amino acids.

To investigate if an intragastric or intravenous amino acid infusion is an appropriate stimulus for the release of a liver-derived factor with the characteristics of glomerulopressin as reported by Uranga and co-workers, we studied the stimulative effect of ultrafiltrate (cut-off approximately 1,000 daltons) of liver vein plasma collected before and after intravenous or intragastric infusion of an amino acid mixture [35]. In studies performed by Uranga and co-workers the stimulative effect of liver vein ultrafiltrate on the contractile tension in gastric fundus muscle was shown to correlate with the stimulative effect on GFR and was used as an index of glomerulopressin activity. We observed that ultrafiltrate of liver vein plasma collected after amino acid infusion had a markedly greater stimulative effect on the contractile tension in the muscle strip than that of liver vein plasma collected before amino acid infusion. To isolate the active compound the ultrafiltrate was subjected to separation by reversed-phase high performance liquid chromatography. The stimulative effect on the fundus muscle strip was confined to one single fraction. By further separation of this fraction, using electrochemical detection high performance liquid chromatography, the active peak was identified as serotonin. The identity of the active substance was confirmed by the observation that the stimulative effect of the ultrafiltrate on the contractile tension of fundus muscle was inhibited by the addition of cyprohepatadine to the incubation medium. Our findings do not agree with the reports of Uranga and co-workers of a liver-derived glucuronide, glomerulopressin, with stimulating effects on gastric smooth muscle and renal hemodynamics [28–30]. Possible explanations for this discrepancy might be that glomerulopressin is not present in man or that in man the concentration of glomerulopressin in liver vein blood collected in the postabsorptive state is below the limit of detection, and that amino acid infusion is not an adequate stimulus for glomerulopressin release from the liver.

Possible Effects of Serotonin on Renal Hemodynamics

Serotonin is a vasoactive substance with complex effects on the renal circulation, ranging from vasoconstriction to secondary vasodilatation [36]. Intravenous infusion of high doses of serotonin in the dog leads to decreases in RBF and GFR [37]. However, infusion of smaller doses of serotonin directly into the renal artery in the dog results in initial marked decrease in RBF followed by a gradual increase which stabilizes well above baseline [38]. This secondary increase RBF is abolished by pretreatment with indomethacin [38]. Results of recent studies show that serotonin stimulates prostaglandin E_2 and prostacyclin synthesis in mesangial cells, suggesting that these vasodilatory prostaglandins may modulate the effect of serotonin on renal hemodynamics [39]. However, whether amino acid-induced release of serotonin from enterochromaffin cells of the gastrointestinal wall may influence renal hemodynamics remains highly speculative. Serotonin is extensively metabolized in the lung [40], and increased release of serotonin from the intestine, leading to a severalfold increase of serotonin in liver vein plasma, may therefore result in just a minor or no increase in the concentration of serotonin in peripheral arterial blood.

References

1 Pitts RF: The effects of infusing glycine and of varying the dietary protein intake on renal hemodynamics in the dog. Am J Physiol 1944;142:355–365.

2 Moustgaard J: Om proteinstoffernes inflydelse paa nyrefunktionen hos hund. Copenhagen, Christensens Forlag, 1948.

3 O'Connor WJ, Summerill RA: The effect of a meal of meat on glomerular filtration rate in dogs at normal urine flows. J Physiol 1976;256:81–91.

4 Bosch JP, Saccaggi A, Lauer A, et al: Renal functional reserve in humnas. Effect of protein intake on glomerular filtration rate. Am J Med 1983;75:943–950.

5 Alvestrand A, Bergström J: Glomerular hyperfiltration after protein ingestion, during glucagon infusion, and in insulin-dependent diabetes is induced by a liver hormone. Lancet 1984;i:195–197.

6 Hostetter TH: Human renal response to a meat meal. Am J Physiol 1986;250:F613–F618.

7 Viberti G, Bognetti E, Wiseman MJ, et al: Effect of protein-restricted diet on renal response to a meat meal in humans. Am J Physiol 1987;253:F388–F393.

8 Brenner BM, Meyer TW, Hostetter TH: Dietary protein intake and the progressive nature of kidney disease: the role of hemodynamically mediated glomerular injury in the pathogensis of progressive glomerular sclerosis in aging, renal ablation, and intrinsic renal disease. N Engl J Med 1982;307:652–659.

9 Lee KE, Summerill RA: Glomerular filtration rate following administration of individual amino acids in conscious dogs. Q J Exp Physiol 1982;67:459–465.

10 Palmore WP: Glucagon and alanine-induced increases of the canine renal glomerular filtration rate. Q J Exp Physiol 1983;68:319–327.

11 Woods LI, Mizelle HL, Hall JE: Role of the liver in renal hemodynamic response to amino acid infusion. Am J Physiol 1987;252:F981–F985.

12 Castellino P, Coda B, DeFronzo RA: Effect of amino acid infusion on renal hemodynamics in humans. Am J Physiol 1986;251:F132–F140.

13 Epstein FH, Brosnan JT, Tange JD, et al.: Improved function with amino acids in the isolated perfused kidney. Am J Physiol 1982;243:F284–F292.

14 Brezis M, Silva P, Epstein FH: Amino acids induce renal vasodilatation in isolated perfused kidney: coupling to oxidative metabolism. Am J Physiol 1984;247:H999–H1004.

15 Meyer TW, Ichikawa I, Zatz R, et al: The renal hemodynamic response to amino acid infusion in the rat. Trans Assoc Am Physiol 1983;96:76–83.

16 Reichlin S: Secretion of somatostatin and its physiological function. J Lab Clin Med 1987;109:320–326.

17 Hirschberg R, Kopple JD: Role of growth hormone in the amino acid-induced acute rise in renal function in man. Kidney Int 1987;32:382–387.

18 Ruilope L, Rodicio J, Miranda B, et al: Renal effects of amino acid infusion in patients with panhypopituitarism. Hypertension 1988;11:557–559.
19 Waldum HL, Sundsfjord JA, Aanstad U, et al: The effect of secretin on renal hemodynamics in man. Scand J Lab Invest 1980;40:475–478.
20 Rocha DM, Faloona GR, Unger RH: Glucagon-stimulating activity of 20 amino acids in dogs. J Clin Invest 1972;51:2346–2351.
21 Johannesen J, Lie M, Kiil F: Effect of glycine and glucagon on glomerular filtration and renal metabolic rates. Am J Physiol 1977;233:F61–F66.
22 Ueda J, Nakanishi H, Miyazaki M, et al: Effects of glucagon on the renal hemodynamics of dogs. Eur J Pharmacol 1977;41:209–212.
23 Parving HH, Noer I, Kehlet H, et al: The effect of short-term glucagon infusion on kidney function in normal man. Diabetologia 1977;13:323–325.
24 Brouhard BH, LeGrone LF, Richards GE, et al: Somatostatin limits rise in glomerular filtration rate after a protein meal. J Pediatr 1987;110:729–734.
25 Claris-Appiani A, Assael BM, Tirelli AS, et al: Lack of glomerular hemodynamic stimulation after infusion of branched-chain amino acids. Kidney Int 1988;33:91–94.
26 Premen AJ, Hall JE, Smith MJ: Postprandial regulation of renal hemodynamics: role of pancreatic glucagon. Am J Physiol 1985;248:F656–F662.
27 Alvestrand A, Bergström J: Glomerular hyperfiltration after protein ingestion, during glucagon infusion, and in insulin-dependent diabetes is induced by a liver hormone. Lancet 1984;i:195–197.
28 Uranga J: The hepatic production of a glomerular pressure substance in the toad (*Bufo arenarum*). Gen Comp Endocrinol 1969;13:179–184.
29 Uranga J: The hepatic production of a glomerular pressure substance in the toad (*Bufo arenarum*). Gen Comp Endocrinol 1969;13:179–184.
30 Uranga J, Fuenzalida R, Rapoport AL, et al: Effect of glucagon and glomerulopressin on the renal function of the dog. Horm Metab Res 1979;11:275–279.
31 Premen AJ: Importance of the liver during glucagon-mediated increases in canine renal hemodynamics. Am J Physiol 1985;249:F319–F322.
32 Dratwa M, Burette A, Van Gossum M, et al: No rise in glomerular filtration rate after protein loading in cirrhotics. Kidney Int 1987;32:S32–S34.
33 Hirschberg R, von Herrath D, Pauls A, et al: No rise in glomerular filtration rate after protein load in severe liver disease. Lancet 1984;ii:1047–1048.
34 Levy M: Inability of glucagon to increase glomerular filtration rate in dogs with experimental cirrhosis and ascites. Can J Physiol Pharmacol 1978;56:511–514.
35 Zimmerman L, Alvestrand A, Bergström J: Elevated concentration of 5-hydroxytryptamine in ultrafiltrate of human liver vein plasma after infusion of amino acids. Acta Physiol Scand 1988;134:399–403.
36 Abboud HE, Dousa TP: Renal metabolism and actions of histamine and serotonin. Miner Electrolyte Metab 1983;9:246–259.
37 Park CS, Chu CS, Park YS, et al: Effect of 5-hydroxytryptamine on renal function in the anesthestized dog. Am J Physiol 1968;214:384–388.
38 Blackshear JL, Orlandi C, Hollenberg K: Serotonin and the renal blood supply: role of prostaglandins and the 5HT-2 receptor. Kidney Int 1986;30:304–310.
39 Knauss T, Abboud HE: Effect of serotonin on prostaglandin synthesis in rat cultured mesangial cells. Am J Physiol 1986;251:F844–F850.
40 Thomas DP, Vane JR: 5-Hydroxytryptamine in the circulation of the dog. Nature 1967;216:355–338.

Anders Alvestrand, MD, Department of Renal Medicine,
Huddinge Hospital, K56, S–141 86 Huddinge (Sweden)

Oldrizzi L, Maschio G, Rugiu C, et al. (eds): The Progressive Nature of Renal Disease: Myths and Facts. Contrib Nephrol. Basel, Karger, 1989, vol 75, pp 26–34

Dietary Components and Progression of Renal Lesions

C. Kleinknecht, D. Laouari, M. Burtin, N. Hinglais
Hôpital Necker Enfants Malades, INSERM U 192, Paris, France

Dietary prescription has been for many years a major concern in the management of chronic renal failure (CRF). In the past it was aimed to limit the accumulation of substances to be excreted by the kidney (osmotic and acid load, waste products of protein metabolism, potassium...) and was begun when the CRF was severe enough for the kidney being unable to cope with normal intakes. Such restrictions have become less essential since renal replacement therapy is easily available, but a new concept emerged recently: the influence of nutritional intakes on the progression of renal lesions which develop in the presence of reduced functional kidney mass [1–3].

It is known that renal lesions develop during aging, in rats as in men, and it seems that similar lesions are accelerated in the presence of reduced renal mass. Their progression depends principally on the amount of functioning renal tissue. They remain mild in aging rats with normal kidneys. They are enhanced after ablation of one kidney, but not sufficiently for end-stage renal disease (ESRD) being reached before natural death occurs from other causes. When renal ablation is more important, as in the 'remnant kidney model' where approximately five sixths of renal mass is removed or destroyed by infarction, the extension of renal lesions results in ESRD. These lesions are not specific, and are glomerular progressive hyalinosis and sclerosis with tubular atrophy and interstitial fibrosis [4]. Experimental studies have shown that other factors than the mass of functional tissue could influence the progression of renal damage. Among them, nutritional factors, and more particularly protein intake [5, 6], have been the most studied, and experimental data suggest that dietetic prescription may be a major point, not only in the late, but also in the early stage of CRF to retard the occurrence of ESRD. The role of dietary components in the progression of lesions resulting from other pathological processes has been little studied.

Food Restriction and Food Excess

Many studies have established that restriction of daily intake of a well-balanced diet markedly prolongs survival, by retarding the occurrence of vascular and tumoral diseases, and completely prevents the development of renal lesions, despite the prolonged life span [7]. Food excess, as observed in hyperphagic rats, is associated with an early development of renal lesions which are prevented by food restriction [8].

Role of Proteins

Amount of Proteins. A lot of previous experiments have stressed that the development of renal lesions during aging was influenced by the protein diet [7, 9]. Bras and Ross [10], for example, decreased the daily protein allotment from 3 to 0.8 g/day while maintaining constant the energy intake in normal rats. They found that the index of renal lesions at time of death decreased from 25 to 10 by reducing protein intake.

Many reports have also shown that development of renal lesions after unilateral nephrectomy was influenced by the protein content of the diet [11, 12]. However neither in aging nor after nephrectomy did these lesions destroy the kidney and result in ESRD before death occurred from usual causes.

After subtotal nephrectomy, Swendseid et al. [13] showed that survival could be modified by the protein content of the diet, but it could not be decided whether death resulted from the progression of lesions or from the 'uremic toxicity', or to what extent the protein content of the diet had influenced appetite and intake of the nutrients.

Some years ago it has been suggested that protein requirement for optimal growth was increased in CRF. To examine this assertion, growth and long-term evolution of growing uremic rats were compared under feeding three different isoenergetic diets differing in their protein content which was 14, 27, and 37% of total energy. In this experiment, proteins were supplied by fish flour which is rich in minerals (calcium, phosphorus and sodium). It was observed that growth was inversely related to the diet protein content (contrarily to what happens in normal rats) and the higher the protein intake, the shorter was the survival despite persistence of normal blood pressure [14]. The remnant kidney taken at the time of spontaneous death showed diffuse renal damage.

A second experiment compared diets offering 7 and 14% of energy as proteins, which were supplied by fish flour. The 7% protein diet caused anorexia and stunting but allowed a markedly prolonged survival [15].

Another experiment compared three different protein diets in adult uremic rats to minimize the possible effects of growth, with proteins supplied by casein so that the intake of all nutrients, including minerals, was identical. Again survival was clearly influenced by protein intake [16].

All these studies were paid little attention until recently, when Hostetter et al. [17] reported that early hemodynamic and morphological changes observed early after subtotal nephrectomy were considerably blunted by feeding a low protein diet, suggesting a possible deleterious effect of hemodynamic adaptive processes.

During the past few years a number of experimental studies in rats have confirmed and emphasized the importance of protein intake [17–21]. In most of these studies, daily food intake was not measured. Since low protein intake usually results in anorexia, it is not always possible to assert that the improvement observed was solely due to proteins. However in two of the experiments quoted [14, 16], the highest protein intake resulted in decreased food intake and accelerated lesions so that any role of other nutrients could be excluded. Finally the role of protein per se in the experimental conditions cannot be denied.

Quality of Proteins. It has been suggested that the nature of the protein used could play a role. Blatherwick [11] compared rats with uninephrectomy fed beaf meat, liver meat, or casein and found differences in progression of renal lesions, but since food intake was not measured differences in food consumption cannot be excluded. Williams et al. [22] observed fewer lesions in uremic rats fed soya protein than in rats fed casein, but soya protein resulted in both lower body weight and decreased urea excretion, suggesting a poor intestinal absorption.

Other authors have found that in adult normal Fisher rats, renal lesions were found at time of spontaneous death in only 7% of rats receiving soya protein, and in 46% of rats receiving the same amount of protein as casein [23]. The main practical problem remains the optimal protein allotment to obtain the maximal kidney preservation while preserving nutritional status, and particularly growth in young animals. To meet this point, semi-synthetic diets have been proposed but they have been surprisingly little studied in animals. In several experiments we observed that diets affording protein as casein, or casein reduced by 50% supplemented with essential amino acids (EAA), resulted in identical food intakes and growth rates, so that the only difference between such two groups was the amount of nonessential amino acid (NEAA) ingested. When an insufficient protein diet (7%) was compared to the same diet supplemented with EAA and to diet affording the minimal requirements for optimal growth (14%) [15], it was observed that EAA addition, while restoring appetite and growth, markedly increased the mortality rate, which was but slightly lower than that of the 14% protein diet fed rats. The difference did not reach significance with the small number of rats studied. In modified experimental conditions however the benefit of reducing only NEAA ingestion was clear [6]: proteins were given separately from the other nutrients, and in agar-gel rich in water, so that uremic rats ingested large amounts of protein. The difference in the amounts of NEAA consumed, which has been 0.6 g/day in the former experiment, reached 1.5 g/day. All 11 rats ingesting whole casein had developed diffuse renal damage within 3 months, whereas 4 of 13 rats receiving reduced amounts of casein supplemented with EAA had diffuse lesions, despite identical energy intake and growth.

The benefit of keto analogue mixtures, where five of the EAA are replaced by their nonnitrogen keto acid (KA), which can be transaminated and transformed in the corresponding EAA in vivo, has not been well established. Barsotti et al. [24] observed a preservation of the remnant kidney in rats fed a very low protein diet (3%) supplemented with such an EAA-KA mixture, compared to rats fed a 20% protein diet, with a trifling though significant difference of weight in adult uremic rats. Whether renal preservation depended on low intake of NEAA, on the replacement of EAA by their KA or on both has not been examined. To our knowledge, no study compared the effects of EAA administration with those of KA administration.

We previously tried to examine this point but the severe anorexia resulting from the KA mixture in the condition used allowed no conclusion regarding KA, although emphasized the complete protection of the kidney in the presence of undernutrition [6, 25]. More recently, we found that EAA-KA mixture with KA as basic amino acid salts was consistent with a satisfactory nutritional status. After 3 months, no difference was found by renal biopsy between rats fed the reference casein diet, or low casein diets supplemented with EAA or with EAA-KA mixture; after 5 months, urinary protein and plasma creatinine tended to be higher with the reference casein diet, but no clear difference existed between the two semisynthetic diets [unpublished data].

Renal Lesions of Other Origin. There is some evidence for a role of proteins on the evolution of renal disorders other than aging and nephron loss, particularly on the immune-mediated nephropathies. In NZB × NZW mice, survival was improved by feeding diets deficient in some amino acids, by restricting protein allotment, and renal lesions were also reduced by a lower protein intake [6]. In experimental nephrotoxic glomerulonephritis, Farr and Smadel [26] observed that mortality diminished when protein diets were reduced from 40 to 18 and 5%. A more recent study observed no renal damage in rats fed a 4% protein diet, diffuse renal lesions in rats fed a 50% protein diet, and intermediate lesions in rats fed a 18% protein diet, although diets were introduced after the introduction of the nephropathy [27]. However the number of studies and the number of animals under study were too few to draw any definite conclusion.

An effect of dietary protein content has been reported in renal lesions following irradiation, diabetes, hypertension, whether genetic or induced by DOCA and salt, and adriamycin induced nephrosis [in ref. 6]. All these results remain to be confirmed in further studies.

Carbohydrates

Carbohydrate-Energy Intake. Carbohydrate (CHO)-energy restriction has been shown to have a dramatic beneficial effect on the lesions of aging [10], of immune diseases [28], of a genetically transmitted nephropathy, and in nephron reduction [29]. Whether these effects result principally of the CHO or of the energy restriction is not known, and there is no evidence that CHO or energy excess has adverse effects. Hyperphagic Zucker rats develop early renal lesions which can be prevented by food restriction, but the relative role of the different nutrients, and the role of the metabolic disturbances existing in this rat stock have been little evaluated.

Carbohydrate Source. While restricting energy as CHO, we observed that restricting glucose was more effective for preservation of the remnant kidney than restricting starch, so that the possibility of a difference in renal adverse effect between mono- and polysaccharides could be raised [29]. However such a difference was not observed in further experiments performed in standard conditions of feeding.

By contrast there is some accumulating evidence for an adverse effect of sucrose. Sucrose feeding is poorly tolerated in uremia. In children there is a clear aversion for high sucrose concentrations in usual foods, compared to normal children [30] and in uremic rats sucrose feeding results in a severe anorexia which was not observed in normal rats [31]. Despite this anorexia leading to food restriction, sucrose-fed rats showed an accelerated death compared to that of rats receiving glucose or starch. In Zucker polyphagic uremic rats, sucrose also resulted in significantly accelerated death compared to rats receiving the same amount of diets containing CHO as glucose or starch [31]. However death could result from ESRD or from other causes, so that the renal adverse effect of sucrose could not be asserted. In uremic lean Zucker rats by contrast, the development of renal lesions was clearly increased by feeding sucrose diet. The mechanism of the effect is not clear: it is known that sucrose-rich diets increase the plasma triglyceride levels, which may play a role in renal deterioration; biochemical changes of the glomerular basement membrane in normal rats fed sucrose-rich diets have been described, and it can be imagined that these changes are enhanced by nephron reduction.

Lipids

It is known that cholesterol-rich diets may cause renal damage. However, data regarding cholesterol in rats cannot be compared to what happens, or could happen, in humans: in rats cholesterol is not the same (HDL and not LDL) and has a different metabolism. In experimental uremia, for example, plasma cholesterol levels parallel plasma creatinine levels, a fact which does not occur in humans.

The main data regarding dietary lipids are the results of diet rich in prostaglandin precursors. Several studies reported that diets rich in fish oil or linoleic acid prevented the deterioration of remnant kidney [32, 33], and/or had a marked beneficial effect on the evolution of blood pressure [33, 34]. However one study concluded to a deleterious effect of a diet rich in eicosapentaenoic acid [35], a result opposite to that of other authors.

A beneficial effect of such diets has also been reported in adriamycin-induced nephrosis [36]. Diets deficient in essential fatty acids were shown to improve immunologically induced renal lesions [37].

Minerals

The role of dietary phosphorus has been the most studied. A diet devoid of phosphorus was claimed to prevent renal deterioration by preventing renal calcifications [38]. In fact, the beneficial effect of this diet seemed mainly mediated by reduced food intake resulting from phosphorus deprivation, and the dramatic calcifications observed, which are quite unusual in the remnant kidney model, were probably artifactual and resulted from the presence of bovin fibrin as a protein source or from the nature of phosphorus salts [39]. It remains that another study showed that low phosphorus intake with low plasma phosphorus levels preserved the remnant kidney [40]. This last experiment however compared rats with low plasma phosphorus levels to rats with high, and not normal, phosphorus levels. From all these experiments it is difficult to decide whether the differences observed resulted from phosphorus load to the kidney, from the presence or absence of a hyperparathyroidism, or from low metabolic activity due to phosphorus deficiency.

Acid Load

High-protein diets increase the amount of ammonia to be excreted. It has been suggested that the amount of ammonia in the kidney could play a role in complement component activation triggering interstitial damage. Whatever the mechanism, supplementation in bicarbonate revealed to be beneficial in the remnant kidney model [41].

Osmotic Load [42, 43]

Some authors have suggested that the increased water reabsorption resulting from high-protein diets could be damaging for the kidney in the presence of severe nephron reduction [42]. Preliminary data tend to show a possible preservative effect of water loading associated to high-protein diets.

Conclusion

An increasing number of nutrients seem to affect the deterioration of the kidney, at least in the remaining kidney model in the rat. There is some evidence for a similar development of renal lesions in dogs, and more importantly in humans, such as demonstrated by the evolution of oligo-meganephronia, where the original condition is nothing but a reduced renal mass. Although none of the numerous studies published on humans demonstrates the protective effect of low-protein diets, because of methologic problems, the evidence can be considered as strong enough to limit protein intake, or at least to avoid the excess usual in developed countries. Limitation of protein implies a decrease in osmotic and acid loads and, in human nutrition, of phosphorus intake. Whether all the nutrients possibly involved in the remnant kidney model also play a role in other conditions, as suggested by some studies, remains to be further evaluated.

Finally it can be suggested that some nutrients affect the oxygen consumption and the metabolic activity of the kidney, such as proteins, energy restriction, osmotic and acid loads, whereas other nutrients, such as sucrose or polyunsaturated acids, could play a role through a different mechanism.

References

1 Klahr S, Buerkert J, Purkerson ML: Role of dietary factors in the progression of chronic renal disease. Kidney Int 1983;24:579–587.

2 Laouari D, Kleinknecht C: The role of nutritional factors in the course of experimental renal failure. Am J Kidney Dis 1985;3:147–156.

3 Kleinknecht C, Laouari D: The influence of dietary components in experimental renal disease in contemporary issues; in Brenner BM, Stein YH, Mitch W (eds): Nephrology, Edinburgh, Churchill-Livingstone, 1986, vol 14; pp 17–35.

4 Waldherr R, Gretz N: Natural course of the development of histological lesions after 5/6 nephrectomy. Contrib Nephrol 1988;60:64–72.

5 Brenner BM, Meyert W, Hostetter TH: Dietary protein intake and the progressive nature of kidney disease. N Engl J Med 1983;307:652–655.

6 Kleinknecht C, Laouari D, Hinglais N: Protein intake and deterioration of renal function in rats: experimental data and hypothetical mechanisms. Contrib Nephrol 1988;60:135–151.

7 Berg BN, Simms HS: Nutrition and longevity in the rat. III. Food restriction beyond 800 days. J Nutr 1961;74:23–32.

8 Kennedy GC: Effects of old age and overnutrition on the kidney. Br Med Bull 1957;13:67–70.

9 Ross MH: Length of life and nutrition in the rat. J Nutr 1961;75:197–210.

10 Bras G, Ross MH: Kidney disease and nutrition in the rat. Toxicol Appl Pharmacol 1964;6:247–262.

11 Blatherwick NR, Medlar EM: Chronic nephritis in rats fed high protein diets. Arch Intern Med 1937;59:572–596.

12 Lalich JJ, Burkholder PM, Paik WC: Protein overload nephropathy in rats with unilateral nephrectomy. Arch Pathol 1975;99:72–79.

13 Swendseid ME, Wang M, Vyhmeister P, et al: Amino acid metabolism in chronically uremic rat. Clin Nephrol 1975;3:240–246.

14 Kleinknecht C, Salusky I, Broyer M, et al: Effect of various protein diets on growth, renal function and survival of uremic rats. Kidney Int 1979;15:534–541.

15 Salusky I, Kleinknecht C, Broyer M, et al: Prolonged renal survival and stunting with protein-deficient diets in experimental uremia. J Lab Clin Med 1981;97:21–30.

16 Laouari D, Kleinknecht C, Gubler MC, et al: Adverse effects of protein on the remnant kidney: dissociation from that of other nutrients. Kidney Int 1983;24(suppl 16):S248–S253.

17 Hostetter TH, Olson JL, Rennke HG, et al: Hyperfiltration in remnant nephrons. A potentially adverse response to renal ablation. Am J Physiol 1981;141:F85–F93.

18 El-Nahas SM, Paraskevakou H, Zoob S, et al: Effect of dietary protein restriction in the development of renal failure after a subtotal nephrectomy in rats. Clin Sci 1983;65:399–600.

19 Hostetter TH, Meyer TW, Rennke HG, et al: Chronic effect of dietary protein in the rats with intact or reduced kidney mass. Kidney Int 1986;30:509–517.

20 Kenner CH, Evan AP, Blomgren P, et al: Effect of protein intake on renal function and structure in partially nephrectomized rats. Kidney Int 1985;27:739–750.

21 Nath KA, Kren SM, Hostetter TH: Dietary protein restriction in established renal injury in the rat. J Clin Invest 1986;78:1199–1205.

22 Williams AJ, Baker FE, Walls J: Effect of varying quantity and quality of dietary protein intake in experimental renal disease in rats. Nephron 1987;46:83–90.

23 Iwasaki K, Gleiser CA, Masoro EJ, et al: The influence of dietary protein source on

longevity and age: related disease processes of Fisher rats. J Gerontol Biochim 1988;43:B5–B12.
24 Barsotti G, Cupisti A, Dani L, et al: Protection of renal function in subtotally nephrectomized rats by dietary therapy. Contrib Nephrol 1986;53:21–30.
25 Laouari D, Kleinknecht C, Dodu C, et al: Nutritional effects of keto-acid-supplemented diets in rats. Contrib Nephrol 1988;60:159–178.
26 Farr LE, Smadel JE: The effects of dietary protein on the course of nephrotoxic nephritis in rats. J Exp Med 1939;70:615–627.
27 Neugarten J, Feiner HD, Schacht RC, et al: Amelioration of experimental glomerulonephritis by dietary protein restriction. Kidney Int. 1983;24:595–601.
28 Fernandes G, Yunis EJ, Good RA: Influence of diet on survival of mice. Proc Natl Acad Sci USA 1976;73:1279–1283.
29 Kleinknecht C, Laouari D, Hinglais N, et al: Role of amount and nature of carbohydrates in the course of experimental renal failure. Kidney Int 1986;30:687–693.
30 Bellisle F, Dartois AM, Kleinknecht C, et al: Perception and preferences for sweet taste in uremic children. 5th Int Congr Nutr Metab Renal Disease. Strasbourg, 1988, abstract, p 15.
31 Laouari D, Kleinknecht C, Burtin M, et al: Adverse effects of sucrose-rich diets in uremic rats. 5th Int Congr Nutr Metab Renal Disease. Strasbourg, 1988, abstract, p 100.
32 Barcelli UO, Weiss M, Pollack VE, et al: Effects of dietary prostaglandin precursor on the progression of experimentally induced chronic renal failure. J Lab Clin Med 1982;100:786–797.
33 Heifets M, Morrissey JJ, Purkerson ML, et al: Effects of dietary lipids on renal function in rats with subtotal nephrectomy. Kidney Int 1987;32:335–341.
34 Izumi Y, Weiner TW, Franco-Saenz R, et al: Effects of dietary linoleic acid on blood pressure and renal function in subtotally nephrectomized animals. Proc Soc Exp Biol Med 1986;183:193–198.
35 Scharschmidt LA, Gibbons NB, McGary L, et al: Effects of dietary fish oil on renal insufficiency in rats with subtotal nephrectomy. Kidney Int 1987;32:700–709.
36 Ito Y, Barcelli U, Yamahita W, et al: Fish oil has beneficial effects on lipids and renal disease of nephrotic rats. Metabolism 1988;37:352–357.
37 Prickett J, Robinson D, Steinberg A: Dietary enrichment with polyunsaturated fatty acid eicosapentaenoic acid prevents proteinuria and prolongs survival in NZB × NZW F1 mice. J Clin Invest 1981;68:556–559.
38 Ibels LS, Alfred AC, Haut L, et al: Preservation of function in experimental renal disease by dietary restriction in phosphate. N Engl J Med 1978;298:122–127.
39 Laouari D, Kleinknecht C, Cournot-Witner G, et al: Beneficial effects of low phosphorus diet in uremic rats: A reappraisal. Clin Sci 1982;63:253–268.
40 Lumlertgul D, Burke TJ, Gillium DM, et al: Phosphate depletion arrests progression of chronic renal failure independent of protein intake. Kidney Int 1986;29:658–666.
41 Nath K, Tolins JP, Hostetter MM, et al: The role of ammonia in progressive renal failure. 5th Int Congr Nutr Metab Renal Disease. Strasbourg, 1988, abstract, p 125.
42 Bouby N, Trinh-Trang-Tan MM, Laouari D, et al: Role of urinary concentration process in the renal effects of high protein intake. Kidney Int 1988;34:4–12.
43 Bankir L, Bouby N, Trinh MM, et al: Possible involvement of antidiuretic hormone and urine concentration in the progression of chronic renal failure. 5th Int Congr Nutr Metab Renal Disease. Strasbourg, 1988, abstract, p 13.

Dr. C. Kleinknecht, INSERM U192, Hôpital Necker, Tour Technique, 6e Etage,
149 rue de Sèvres, F–75743 Paris Cédex 15 (France)

Oldrizzi L, Maschio G, Rugiu C, et al. (eds): The Progressive Nature of Renal Disease: Myths and Facts. Contrib Nephrol. Basel, Karger, 1989, vol 75, pp 35–44

Protection of Residual Renal Function by Different Dietary Regimens in Subtotally Nephrectomized Rats

G. Barsotti, A. Cupisti, E. Morelli, F. Ciardella, G. Schipani, S. Giovannetti

Reparto di Nefrologia, Clinica Medica 1, Università di Pisa, Italia

The progressive renal insufficiency following subtotal nephrectomy or experimental glomerulopathies in rats can be prevented by the restriction of protein intake [1, 2]. In these models of renal diseases the protection of the remnant kidney tissue has been obtained at the price of stunting [3, 4] or weight [5]. Recently we prevented the onset and the progression of nephropathy following subtotal nephrectomy in rats by using a low-protein, low-phosporus diet, supplemented with essential amino acids and ketoanalogues [6]. Similar results have been obtained in five-sixths nephrectomized rats fed a normal protein diet supplemented with dihydroxyaluminum monocetate, a potent phosphate binder that induces phosphate depletion [7].

The first aim of the present investigation is to evaluate the possibility of an effective protection of the residual renal function by using a low-protein, low-phosphorus diet supplemented with essential amino acids (EAA) and ketoanalogues (KA), without inducing malnutrition or stunting, in subtotally nephrectomized rats with already established severe renal failure. Secondarily, to assess if the phosphorus dietary restriction alone (with a normal protein intake) exerts the same effects on renal function and nutritional status.

Materials and Methods

The experimental design has been performed in two different ways:

'Treatment' of Severe and Progressive Renal Failure with a Low-Protein, Low-Phosphorus Supplemented Diet

Thirty Wistar adult male rats underwent five-sixths nephrectomy in two stages: first, the two poles of the left kidney were surgically ablated, and the residual renal cortex was cauterized with a hot stylus in five points [4]. Ten days later the right kidney was removed.

Table 1. Components of the diets

	LSD	LSLPiD	SD g/100 g
Carbohydrates	67	67	62
Lipids	3	3	20
Proteins	20.5	20.5	3.3[2]
EAA and KA supplemented	0.0	0.0	7.5
Calcium	1.1	1.1	1.1
Phosphorus	0.98	0.21	0.27
Sodium	0.002	0.002	0.002
Potassium	0.85	0.85	0.85
Total nitrogen	3.3	3.3	1.1
Kilocalories/100 g	376	376	433

[1]Mostly as ovalbumin. [2]Only from vegetables.

During a 3-month period all rats were maintained on a low-sodium, normal protein and phosphorus diet (LSD, table 1). All rats developed a severe, progressive renal failure and significant proteinuria. Eight of them died. The 22 surviving rats were then randomized to: *LSD group (controls)* – ten rats that continued the LSD; *SD group* – 12 rats that changed to the SD. The SD is a low-protein, low-phosphorus diet, supplemented with EAA and KA (table 1).

The EAA and KA supplements were identical to those used in chronic uremics [8]. The sodium content of LSD and SD is identical and very low, while the protein (exclusively from vegetables) and phosphorus content is much lower (table 1).

The 8 surviving rats of the SD group were sacrificed 120 days after randomization when they still were in a good condition. The 6 surviving rats of the LSD group were sacrificed 60 days after randomization when the death from uremia appeared impending.

'Treatment' of Progressive and Severe Chronic Uremia with a Low-Sodium, Low-Phosphorus Diet

Twenty-four male adult Wistar rats were subtotally nephrectomized as above and submitted to LSD. Three months later the 16 surviving uremic rats were randomly allocated into two groups: *LSD group* (controls) – 8 rats which continued LSD (table 1); low-sodium, low-phosphorus diet (*LSLPiD*) *group* – 8 rats which changed to a low-phosphorus, normal protein diet. The sodium and protein content of LSLPiD was identical to the LSD, while the phosphorus was much lower, and similar to the SD (table 1). The 6 surviving rats of both groups were sacrificed 2 months after randomization.

We studied the following parameters: creatinine clearance (ml/min · 10^2, CrCl), urinary protein loss (mg/day, UPr), urinary phosphorus (mg/day, UPi) and urinary urea nitrogen (mg/day, UUN) excretion, body weight (BW, g), UUN/BW ratio (mg/g/day), light microscopy of the remnant kidney tissue and mortality. CrCl, UPr, UPi and UUN were measured every 30 days by using metabolic cages for 24-hour urine collection (from 9 a.m. to 9 a.m. of the next day). The blood samples were drawn at the end of urine collection period, while the rats were under ether anesthesia. Simultaneously the BW was measured. sCr, UCR, UPi and UU were

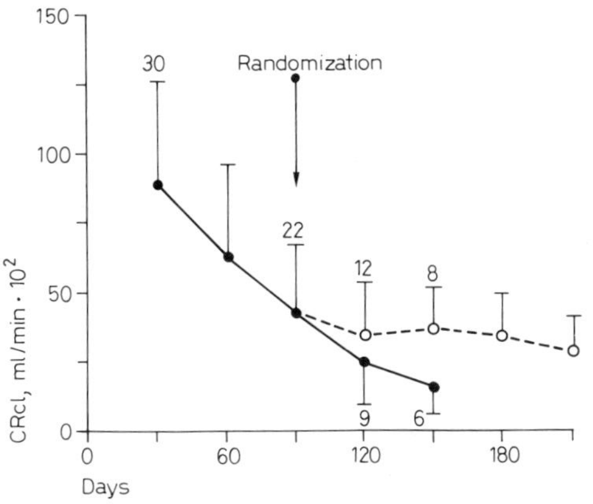

Fig. 1. The behavior of CrCl in rats before and after randomization into the study group (○) and the control group (●). Mean ± SD.

determined with a standard auto-analyzer. UPr was measured with the Ponceau-red method. For the kidney tissue specimens we used three different staining techniques: periodic acid-Schiff (PAS), hematoxylin-eosin (HE) and von Kossa specific staining for calcium, deposits.

In order to determine the severity and the activity of histological damage we employed the following renal pathology screening system: *(a) glomerular lesions* – endothelial-mesangial proliferation, epithelial and fibrous crescents, capillary loop thrombosis, sclerohyalinosis and glomerulo-capsular synechiae; *(b) tubular-interstitial lesions* – tubular cell degeneration and necrosis, tubular dilation and atrophy, interstitial cellular infiltration and fibrosis, and calcium-phosphate deposits; *(c) vascular alterations* – vasculitis, arteriolosclerosis with wall thickening or occlusion.

All these lesions were expressed as the percent of the renal structures found in five different microscopial fields. Proliferation, crescents, thrombosis, cellular infiltrates, cellular degeneration and necrosis were defined as *active lesions*. Fibrosis, sclerohyalinosis, tubular cell atrophy and tubule dilatation, arteriolar or arterial sclerosis were considered *chronic, stable lesions*.

The results were expressed as mean ± SD. p values lower than 0.05 were considered statistically significant. The statistical evaluation of the results was performed by the Student's 't' test for unpaired data.

Results

'Treatment' of Severe and Progressive Renal Failure with a Low-Protein, Low-Phosphorus Supplemented Diet

Creatinine Clearance. The rate of CrCl decreased along the time during the 3-month period of LSD. This decline of the residual renal function continued in those rats which followed LSD after randomization. The rats which changed to the SD showed a relatively stable CrCl lasting 4 months after randomization (fig. 1).

1
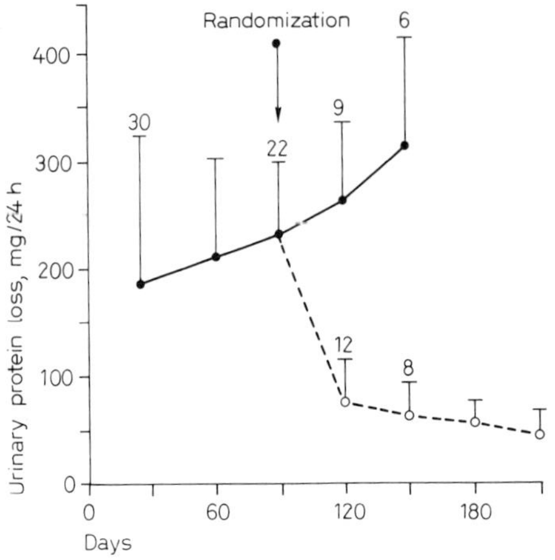

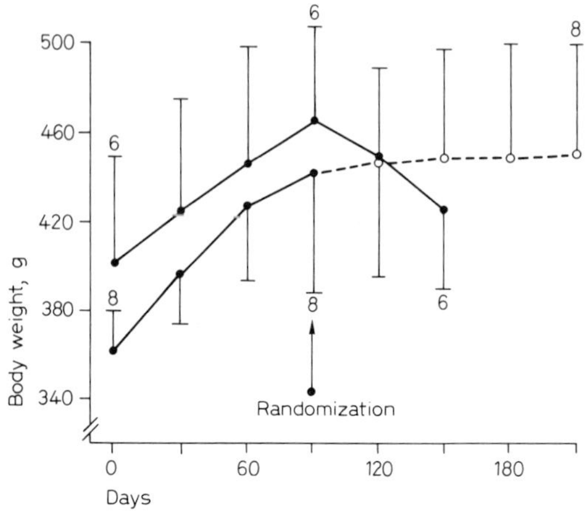

2

Fig. 2. The urinary protein loss before and after randomization into the control group (●) and the study group (○). Mean ± SD.

Fig. 3. The BW changes in the control rats on LSD (●) and in rats of the experimental group (○). Mean ± SD.

Urinary Protein Loss. UPr increased progressively during the pre-randomization period, reaching the mean value of 228.4 ± 71.1 mg/day. It further increased in the LSD group after randomization, reaching a mean value of 312.4 ± 100.6 mg/day in the 6 rats surviving until sacrifice (fig. 2). In the rats switched to the SD after randomization the UPr fell significantly, and reached the mean value of 47.2 ± 22.8 mg/day at the end of the experiment (fig. 2).

Body Weight Changes. As shown in figure 3, the BW increased progressively during the follow-up period before randomization, when all rats followed LSD. After randomization, the BW of control rats on LSD decreased from 468.4 ± 54.2 to 427.1 ± 37.6 g ($p < 0.05$). The rats which changed from LSD to SD showed an increase of BW from 442.6 ± 60.2 to 459.0 ± 51.7 g (p: n.s.). The mean overall weight *gain* in the SD group after randomization was 7.4 ± 11.4 g, while the LSD group had a mean weight *loss* of 48.8 ± 12.6 g.

Urinary Urea Nitrogen/Body Weight Ratio. The UUN/BW ratio changed from 0.457 ± 0.087 to 0.624 ± 0.120 mg/g/day in the LSD group after randomization ($p < 0.001$). In the rats of the SD group this index, calculated one month after randomization (0.113 ± 0.027 mg/g/day) and at

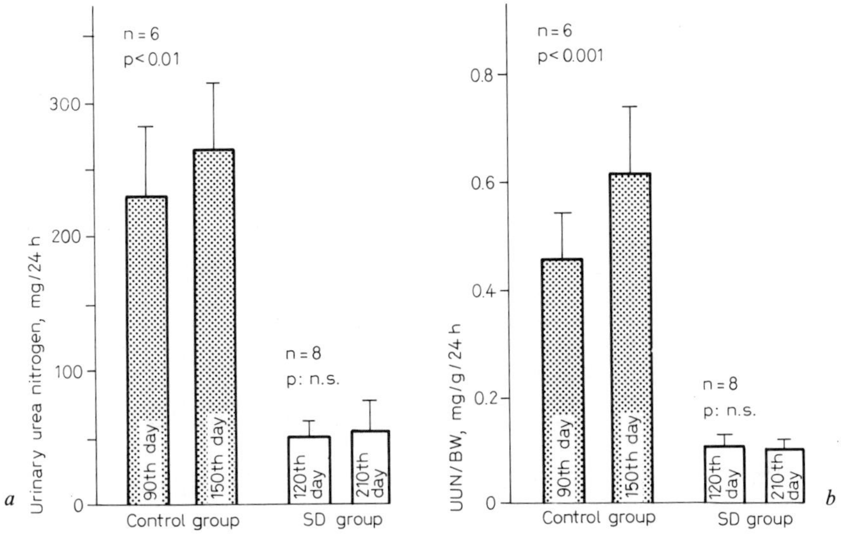

Fig. 4. The changes of the daily UUN excretion *(a)* and of the UUN/BW ratio *(b)*, measured at the 90th and 150th days in controls on LSD (dotted columns) and at the 120th and 210th days in rats on SD (with the columns). Mean ± SD.

the end of the study period (0.111 ± 0.012), did not change (fig. 4). The low values of UUN in the SD group accounts for the very low protein supply of the SD.

Light Microscopy Findings. The results are summarized in table 2. The rats of the LSD group showed a very high incidence of *active* and *chronic* lesions, such as endothelial and mesangial proliferation, epithelial crescents, segmental or global glomerular sclerohyalinosis, glomerulocapsular synechiae, with capillary loop thrombosis, interstial infiltrates, tubular cell degeneration and tubule dilatation, calcium phosphate deposits and thickening of arteriolar walls with lumen reduction or obliteration. The abnormalities observed in the remnant kidney tissue of the SD group were much less severe, and predominantly *chronic*. Segmental glomerular sclerosis and glomerulocapsular synechiae were present in all rats of this group, while mesangial proliferations and crescents were absent. As shown in table 2, the tubular, interstitial and vascular lesions were much less severe and frequent than in the LSD group.

Mortality. During the 3-month period before randomization 8 rats died. Among the 12 rats of the SD group 4 died 2 months after

Table 2. Histological findings in remnant kidney tissue in surviving rats at the sacrifice, expressed as a percent of frequency

LSLPiD	Control on LSD (n = 12)	Rats on SD (n = 8)	Rats on LSLPiD (n = 8)
Glomeruli			
Sclerosis	+++(32)	−	+++(30)
	++(60)	++(38)	++(54)
	−(8)	−(62)	−(16)
Mesangial proliferation	+++(18)	−	+++(16)
	++(82)	++(10)	++(76)
	−(0)	−(90)	−(8)
Crescents	+++(6)	−	+++(4)
	++(40)	−	++(32)
	−(54)	−(100)	−(64)
Thrombosis	+++(25)	−	+++(22)
	++(25)	++(20)	++(36)
	−(50)	−(80)	−(42)
Tubules			
Degeneration	+++(25)	−	+++(30)
	++(20)	++(40)	++(45)
	−(55)	−(60)	−(75)
Atrophy	+++(50)	+++ (8)	+++(55)
	++(30)	++(25)	++(30)
	−(20)	−(68)	−(15)
Dilatation	+++(32)	+++(7)	+++(42)
	++(34)	++(40)	++(40)
	−(34)	−(43)	−(18)
Interstitium			
Infiltration	+++(30)	−	+++(36)
	++(60)	++(55)	++(50)
	−(10)	−(54)	−(14)
Fibrosis	+++(32)	−	+++(36)
	++(20)	++(40)	++(24)
	−(48)	−(60)	−(40)
Calcium-phosphate deposits	+++(26)	−	−
	++(60)	++(10)	++(18)
	−(14)	−(90)	−(82)
Arteries			
Wall thickening	+++(25)	+++(12)	+++(30)
	++(65)	++(20)	++(62)
	−(10)	−(68)	−(8)
Occlusion	+++(18)	+++(8)	+++(10)
	++(12)	++(10)	++(12)
	−(70)	−(82)	−(78)

+++ = Severe and diffuse lesions; ++ = mild and focal lesions; − = absence of lesions. Percentages are given in parentheses.

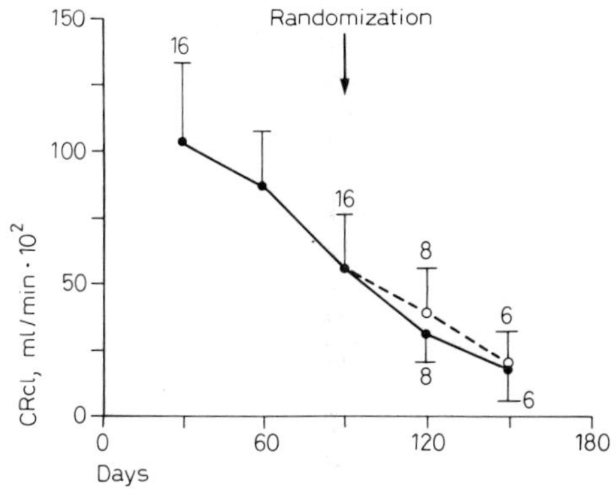

Fig. 5. CrCl changes in control rats on LSD (●) and in the study group on LSLPiD (○). Mean ± SD.

randomization and the remaining 8 were sacrificed 2 months later. The overall mortality in the SD group was 33% during the 4-month period after randomization. Four rats out of the 10 rats which continued LSD died in the first month after randomization, and the surviving 6 were sacrificed 20 days later when clearly they were going to die spontaneously from uremia. The overall mortality in the LSD group was 40% in 60 days.

'Treatment' of Severe and Progressive Renal Failure with a Low-Sodium, Low-Phosphorus Diet

Creatinine Clearance. CrCl decreased with time during the pre-randomization period, reaching the mean value of 56.3 ± 19.4 ml/min 3 months after the five-sixths nephrectomy. After randomization CrCl continued to decline progressively both in the LSD and LSLPiD group. In the 6 surviving rats of the LSD group at the end of experiment the CrCl was identical to the 6 surviving rats of the LSLPiD group (fig. 5).

Urinary Protein Loss. UPr increased progressively in all rats during the 3-month period before randomization, reaching the mean value of 264.1 ± 83.7 mg/day (fig. 6). After randomization there was a reduction of UPr in both LSD and LSLPiD groups, probably because of the progressive reduction of renal function. At the end of the study, UPr was 215.0 ± 53.3 mg/day in the 6 surviving rats of the LSLPiD group and 185.5 ± 78.2 mg/day in the LSD group (p = n.s, fig. 6).

Body Weight Changes. BW decreased in both the LSD and LSLPiD groups after randomization, as appears in figure 7. The BW loss was due to

6 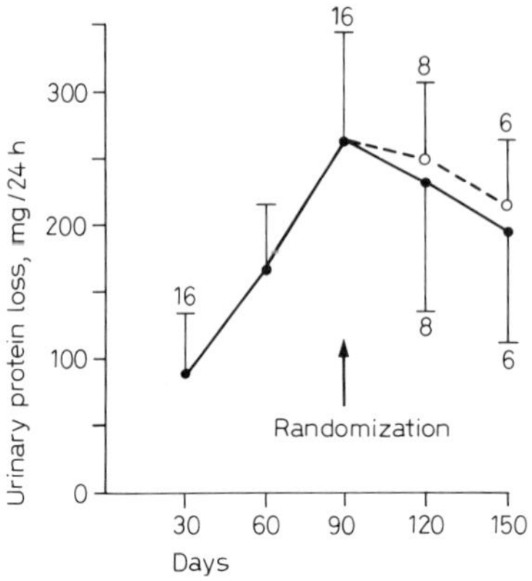

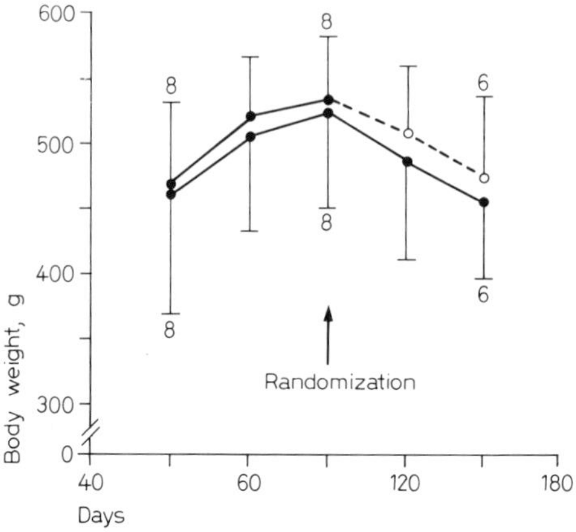 7

Fig. 6. The daily urinary protein loss in controls on LSD (●) and in rats which changed to the LSLPiD (○) after randomization. Mean ± SD.

Fig. 7. The behavior of body weight in control rats following LSD (●) and in rats shifted to LSLPiD after randomization (○). Mean ±SD.

the progressing uremia that induced anorexia. At the sacrifice, the BW in LSD surviving rats was 454.2 ± 51.1 g and in the LSPiD group it was 476.2 g (p = n.s., fig. 7).

Mortality. During the 3-month period before randomization, 8 rats died. The mortality after randomization was identical in the two studied groups (25%).

Light Microscopy Findings. The light microscopical findings found in the remnant kidney tissue of the sacrificed rats at the end of the experiment are summarized in table 2. The feature of the LSD group was identical to that found in the LSD group of the previous experiment, and quite similar to that found in the LSLPiD group. The incidence of interstitial calcium phosphate deposits in this group is very low, as compared to that found in the LSD group.

Discussion

This study clearly demonstrates that the SD exerts a protection of the remnant kidney tissue and residual renal function in rats with severe chronic renal failure. In fact, we observed an almost complete stabilization of CrCl in the SD group after randomization, as compared with the progressive decline found in the LSD group. The lower mortality from uremia may be regarded as a direct consequence of this protective effect of SD.

The impressive reduction of daily urinary protein loss in rats shifted to the SD probably exerts a critical role in such a protection. In our previous 'prevention' experiment, in which SD was started immediately after the five-sixths nephrectomy, we prevented the severe proteinuria and the typical histological abnormalities following subtotal nephrectomy in rats [6]. Severe proteinuria is known to be harmful to the kidney [9–11]. In addition, it has been suggested that circulating protein deposition within the mesangial region may cause an expansion of this area, inducing mesangial cell proliferation and enhanced production of matrix [12, 13].

The hemodynamic mechanisms whereby the glomerular filtration rate increases in rats with five-sixths nephrectomy are well documented by micropunture studies [14, 15]. Hyperfiltration in remnant nephrons is reduced by the dietary protein restriction [16, 17], and this reduction is probably another important cause of the protective effect exerted by SD.

The histological results are in agreement with these findings. The predominant lesions found in the SD group at the end of the study are typically 'chronic', and probably represent the evolution to sclerosis of 'active processes' developed in the course of the pre-randomization period. This clearly proves that the 'active' processes, leading to terminal uremia after subtotal nephrectomy, are strongly hindered by SD.

The nutritional status is well protected by SD, as demonstrated by the slight increase of BW after randomization, whereas the BW of control rats on LSD decreases markedly during the 60-day period after randomization. The progressive uremia, causing both anorexia and catabolism, accounts for this finding in control rats.

The occurrence of a catabolic status in control rats following LSD after randomization is revealed by the increase of UUN simultaneously with a significant decrease of food intake and BW. In contrast, the UUN/BW ratio in rats following SD decreased markedly after randomization, as expected from the very low-protein dietary intake, and did not increase during the 4-month study period after randomization.

A low-phosphorus intake without any protein dietary restriction does not exert protective effect on remnant kidney tissue, as demonstrated by the histological findings in rats of the LSLPiD group, the only difference consisting in a less prevalence of interstitial calcium-phosphate deposits. The LSLPiD failed to protect the residual renal function in rats with severe and progressive CRF, as it appears from the behavior of CrCl plotted against time, quite similar in LSD and LSLPi group. The LSLPiD clearly does not induce phosphate depletion (Lumlertgul), and its phosphorus content is higher than other very low-phosphorus regimens previously employed to retard progression of injury in the remnant kidney (Ibels).

References

1 El Nahas AM, Paraskevakou H, Zoob S, et al: Effect of dietary protein on the development of renal failure after subtotal nephrectomy in rats. Clin Sci 1983;65:399–406.

2 Neugarten J, Feiner HD, Schact RG, et al: Amelioration of experimental glomerulonephritis by dietary protein restriction. Kidney Int 1983;24:595–601.

3 Salusky I, Kleinknect C, Boyer M, et al: Prolonged renal survival and stunting with protein-deficient diets in experimental uremia. J Lab Clin Med 1981;91:21–30.

4 Wang M, Vyhmeister, I, Kopple JD, et al: Effect of protein intake on weight gain and plama amino acid levels in uremic rats. Am J Physiol 1976;5:1455–1459.

5 Okuda S, Motomura S, Sanai T, et al: Effects of different levels of protein intake on renal deterioration and nutritional state in the experimental renal disease. Clin Sci 1987;73:33–39.

6 Barsotti G, Cupisti A, Dani L, et al.: The prevention of the progressive renal failure in subtotally nephrectomized rats following a low-protein, low-phosphorus diet supplemented with essential aminoacids and ketoanalogues. Contrib Nephrol 1986;53:21–30.

7 Lumlertgul D, Burke TJ, Gillum DM, et al.: Phosphate depletion arrests progression of chronic renal failure independent of protein intake. Kidney Int 1986;29:658–666.

8 Barsotti G, Guiducci A, Ciardella F, et al: Effects on renal function of a low-nitrogen diet supplemented with essential aminoacids and ketoanalogues and of hemodialysis and free protein supply in patients with chronic renal failure. Nephron 1981;27:113–117.

9 Robson AM, Mor J, Root ER, et al: Mechanism of proteinuria in non glomerular disease. Kidney Int 1979;16:416–422.

10 Glasser RJ, Velosa JA, Michael AF: Experimental model of focal sclerosis. I. Relationship to protein excretion in aminonucleoside nephrosis. Lab Invest 1977;36:519–526.

11 Velosa JA, Kolley KE, Torres VE, et al: Significance of proteinuria on the outcome of renal function in patients with focal segmental glomerular sclerosis. Mayo Clin Proc 1983;58:568–577.

12 Couser WG, Stilmant MM: Mesangial lesions and focal glomerulosclerosis in the agin rats. Lab Invest 1975;33:491–501.

13 Grond J, Schilthuius MS, Koudstall J, et al: Mesangial function and glomerular sclerosis in rats after unilateral nephrectomy. Kidney Int 1982;22:338–343.

14 Kaufman JM, Siegel NJ, Hayslett JP: Functional and hemodynamic adaptation to progressive renal ablation. Circ Res 1975;36:286–293.

15 Hostetter TH, Olson JL, Rennke HG, et al: Hyperfiltration in remnant nephrons: a potentially adverse response to renal ablation. Am J Physiol 1981;241:F85–F93.

16 Brenner BM, Meyer TW, Hostetter TH: Dietary protein intake and the progressive nature of kidney disease: The role of hemodynamically mediated glomerular injury in the pathogenesis of progressive glomerular sclerosis in aging, renal ablation and intrinsic renal disease. N Engl J Med 1982;307:652–659.

17 Hostetter TH, Meyer TW, Rennke HG, et al: Chronic effects of dietary protein in the rat with intact and reduced renal mass. Kidney Int 1986;30:509–517.

G. Barsotti, MD, Reparto di Nefrologia, Clinica Medica 1,
Università di Pisa, I–56100 Pisa (Italy)

Oldrizzi L, Maschio G, Rugiu C, et al. (eds): The Progressive Nature of Renal Disease: Myths and Facts. Contrib Nephrol. Basel, Karger, 1989, vol 75, pp 45–59

Filtration Surface Area, Salt Intake and Hypertension

Barry M. Brenner[a], *Sharon Anderson*[b]

[a]Renal Divison, Department of Medicine, Brigham and Women's Hospital, and [b]Harvard Center for the Study of Kidney Disease, Harvard Medical School, Boston, Mass., USA

Development of the Hypothesis

Abnormalities in renal sodium handling have been linked to the pathogenesis of experimental and human essential hypertension. In 1963, Ledingham and Cohen [1] proposed that hypertension was initiated by expansion of extracellular fluid and plasma volume, which in turn cause a rise in central venous and right heart pressures, an increase in cardiac output due to the Starling effect, and finally a rise in blood pressure. Natriuresis and diuresis induced by the rise in blood pressure prevent further expansion of extracellular fluid volume (ECV). Thereafter, in the chronic phase, total peripheral resistance rises, with a return of cardiac output to normal, thus changing from high cardiac output-mediated hypertension to a high peripheral resistance form of chronic hypertension. Similar reasoning led others [2] to postulate that certain individuals have an unknown renal defect that requires a higher renal perfusion pressure to excrete the increased load of salt and water, thus rendering these individuals susceptible to the development of hypertension. Cross-transplantation experiments, in which kidneys transplanted from hypertension-prone animals induced hypertension in previously normotensive animals [3, 4], while placement of a kidney from a normotensive donor into a previously hypertensive rat [3, 4] or human [5] recipient restored blood pressure to more normal levels, also lent credence to the important role of the kidney in the genesis of hypertension.

Guyton et al. [6] extended this concept by suggesting that hypertension is characterized by abnormalities in the pressure-natriuresis phenomenon. According to this formulation, in the face of an elevated sodium intake, increased arterial pressure serves to augment renal function and sodium excretion, thereby restoring sodium balance. This feedback mechanism serves to stabilize arterial pressure, albeit at a raised level, because increases in pressure augment sodium and water excretion, thereby preventing further expansion of ECV. Arterial hypertension is the biological price, however, insofar as the kidneys require a higher than normal perfusion pressure to maintain near-normal extracellular fluid volume homeostasis.

Altered renal hemodynamics, reduced ability to excrete sodium, and arterial hypertension also characterize the adaptive response to a decrease in the number of functioning nephrons. Whether acquired as a result of intrinsic renal disease or following surgical renal ablation, reduced nephron number almost invariably gives rise to systemic arterial hypertension. *These observations, together with the evidence described below, lead us to postulate that essential hypertension may at least in part be due to a decreased filtration surface area, due to a congenital reduction in the number of nephrons and/or a congenital decrease in filtration surface area per glomerulus.* A decrease in filtration surface area may lead to renal sodium retention, and thus to systemic hypertension. Systemic hypertension then leads to glomerular capillary hypertension and eventual glomerular sclerosis, which in turn further decreases the surface area available for filtration, perpetuating a vicious cycle. An inherited reduction in filtration surface area may also explain the highly variable rates of expression and progression of human renal disease, in that the hemodynamic burden (i.e. glomerular and systemic hypertension) may render affected individuals less able to sustain renal function after initial injury than those endowed at birth with a greater number of nephrons.

Clinically, inborn deficits in nephron number are associated with the development of hypertension. In the extreme case of oligomeganephronia, a rare form of renal dysgenesis characterized by a reduction in nephron number to only 20–25% of normal (with striking glomerular and tubule enlargement), hypertension, progressive glomerular sclerosis and eventual chronic renal failure are the rule [7, 8]. More common is unilateral renal agenesis, which occurs in approximately 1:1,000 births [9, 10]. This entity is now recognized to lead to early development of hypertension and proteinuria and, in some cases, to end-stage renal failure [11, 12]. Hypertension also supervenes when a comparable reduction in nephron number occurs later in life as a consequence of ablative surgery, does not markedly impair overall renal function appreciably, at least initially, and usually leaves behind an entirely normal kidney [13]. Long-term studies of human subjects who have donated a kidney for transplantation are now becoming available, and indicate that although renal function is well maintained in the majority of donors for up to two decades, loss of one kidney may enhance the risk of hypertension and proteinuria when compared to age- and sex-matched controls [13–15].

Each human kidney has been estimated to contain approximately 800,000–1,000,000 nephrons [16, 17]. However, the nephron population ranges from as low as 600,000 to as high as 1,200,000. At least half the population lies between 800,000 and 1,100,000; fewer than 10% lie above this range, whereas as many as 40% may fall below 800,000 nephrons per kidney [16]. No new nephrons are formed after birth, and the number of functioning glomeruli tends to decrease after age 40, a consequence of normal aging [18].

Are individuals born with nephron numbers in the low end of the distribution range at risk for the development of essential hypertension? Hayman et al. [19], in a study of patients with and without renal disease, found systolic blood pressure to be above 150 mm Hg in individuals with less than 700,000 glomeruli per kidney, suggesting that when glomerular number is reduced to this level (about 30% below the median), there is 'some change associated with the presence of elevated blood pressue'. *We suggest that this 'change' is the low nephron number per se.* It is tempting to speculate that those individuals whose congenital nephron numbers fall toward the lower end of the frequency distribution curve constitute the well-described populations or population subsets that exhibit enhanced susceptibility to the development of essential hypertension. By analogy, those individuals with more than 110% of the median number of nephrons may represent the percentage of the population with blood pressures at the lower end of the normal range. Individuals with nephron numbers near the median (800,000–1,100,000) are more likely to exhibit systemic pressures within the normal range. However, when nephron number falls to about 75% of the median value, borderline hypertension is reached, and individuals with nephron numbers below 700,000 are considered to exhibit overt systemic hypertension.

Increased susceptibility to hypertension may also result from a decrease in filtration surface area when nephron number is normal, but the filtration surface area per glomerulus is reduced. Glomerular diameter, an indirect measure of the surface area available for filtration, varies as much as threefold in infancy, and follows a normal distribution pattern in adult kidneys [20]. Glomerular capillary basement membrane surface area, a more direct reflection of net filtration surface area, also varies as much as threefold in normal kidneys [17]. Thus, a decreased filtration surface area per glomerulus may contribute to hypertension even in the presence of a normal number of nephrons.

Nephron Number and Hypertension: Experimental Evidence

Experimentally, a clear association between glomerular number, dietary sodium intake, and incidence of hypertension has been documented.

Removal of 70% or more of functioning renal mass in the rat leads to systemic and glomerular hypertension, with increased plasma volumes [21] and low plasma renin levels [22]. Indeed, with this degree of renal ablation, hypertension is observed even in the absence of a high sodium intake [23]. With lesser reduction in nephron number, however, as in the case of uninephrectomy, hypertension usually does not develop in rats unless the diet is rich in sodium [24]. Koletsky and Goodsitt [25] found that by increasing dietary sodium content, hypertension could be induced in 100% of rats with 75% nephrectomy after 2 weeks, in 94% of uninephrectomized rats after 4 months, and in 66% of aging rats with two intact kidneys after 8 months.

Increased sodium intake enhances susceptibility to hypertension in certain 'salt-sensitive' hypertensive rat strains, even in the absence of surgical reduction in renal mass. As compared to their respective salt-resistant, normotensive counterparts, rats of the Dahl S and Holtzman salt-sensitive strains exhibit higher values for systemic arterial pressure [26, 27]. Of note, these salt-sensitive strains are associated with a 15% congenital reduction in glomerular number as well as a reduction in the glomerular ultrafiltration coefficient [27], suggesting that decreased filtration surface area per se predisposes to an enhanced susceptibility to salt-sensitive hypertension. Indeed, inborn reductions in nephron number may also lead to systemic hypertension in the absence of a high sodium intake. For example, adult rats of the Milan hypertensive strain have been shown to possess 17% fewer glomeruli, on average, than do their normotensive counterpart, the Milan normotensive strain [28]. Similarly, a reduction in glomerular number has been documented in hypertensive rats of the Munich-Wistar-Fromter strain as compared to their normotensive Han/Wistar controls [29, 30]. Blood pressure is lower, and glomerular numbers 22% higher, in PVG/c rats than in their Wistar controls [31]. In the spontaneously hypertensive rat (SHR), glomerular numbers are slightly, but not significantly, lower than in normotensive Wistar-Kyoto (WKY) rats [32], implying that other renal sodium excretory defects may conspire with this more subtle reduction in nephron number to predispose to systemic hypertension. However, prehypertensive SHR exhibit values for the glomerular capillary ultrafiltration coefficient which are lower than those in WKY, suggesting that filtration surface area, and/or the permeability properties of the filtering capillary, are lower in the SHR [33].

Sodium and Hypertension

Dietary sodium excess is associated with an increased incidence of essential hypertension [34, 35]. Alternatively, populations which ingest less than 30 mEq/day of sodium exhibit virtually no hypertension, and no rise in blood pressure with aging [36]. Some essential hypertensives exhibit blood pressure sensitivity to alterations in sodium intake, an effect detected as early as the first few months of life [37].

Susceptibility to development of essential hypertension is clearly an inherited trait. The risk of hypertension increases dramatically when both parents are hypertensive [38], but this association does not necessarily distinguish between hereditary and shared environmental factors. More convincing evidence for a genetic basis comes from observations within families, including observations of a stronger correlation between identical twins than between fraternal twins or siblings [39], and lack of correlation between parents and adopted children [40]. In addition to a substantial hereditary contribution to baseline blood pressure values, there is a compelling familial resemblance in sodium sensitivity of blood pressure between parents and offspring [41]. Normotensive first-degree relatives of patients with essential hypertension exhibit higher basal blood pressures, and reduced ability to excrete a sodium load, as compared to subjects with no family history of hypertension [42]. Moreover, normotensive teenagers with one hypertensive parent exhibit a rise in blood pressure when subjected to a high sodium intake, whereas normotensive teenagers born of normotensive parents do not [43]. These observations point strongly to an inherited renal abnormality in the pathogenesis of essential hypertension.

There may also be a genetic component to the development of hypertension in humans with a solitary kidney. Renal transplant recipients of a kidney from a normotensive donor with a family history of hypertension exhibit higher values of blood pressure, and require more antihypertensive therapy, than do recipients of grafts from normotensive donors with no family history of hypertension [44] and these recipients tend to show significant increases in blood pressure during acute rejection episodes. Thus, susceptibility to hypertension is conferred not only by transplantation of a kidney from a hypertensive donor, but even by transplantation of a kidney from a normotensive donor with a family history of hypertension. *Do such kidneys contain less filtration surface area (i.e. fewer glomeruli) than those from donors with no such family history?*

Since only a minority of the general population is hypertensive, it seems clear that sodium intake contributes to the development of hypertension only in individuals with a genetic or congenital susceptibility that allows the development of hypertension even in the face of a 'normal' sodium intake. An inherited decrease in nephron number (or filtration surface area), leading to a diminished capacity to excrete a normal sodium load, could constitute the underlying pathogenetic determinant of salt-sensitive essential hypertension in these subjects. Thus, variability in nephron number, with subsequent heterogeneity in blood pressure responses to increased sodium intake, may explain the observed variability in arterial pressures at varying levels of sodium intake. Those individuals whose nephron number is in the middle of the normal distribution (i.e. 100% of 'normal') exhibit relative blood pressure insensitivity to increases (or decreases) in sodium intake, so that a blood pressure increment is seen only with extreme dietary excess, if at all. Those whose nephron number exceeds the median (over 100% of normal) exhibit even lower ambient blood pressures on an average salt intake, and little if any change with extremes of sodium intake. In those subjects with nephron numbers in the lower end of the distribution range, however, lesser increases in sodium intake are believed to be required to raise blood pressure. At the lower end of the nephron number scale, as in patients with advanced renal disease, the ability to modulate sodium excretion is limited, so that greater increases in arterial pressure are required to maintain external balance even at relatively moderate dietary sodium intake.

Though largely unexplored, inborn deficits in nephron number could contribute to the observed differences in susceptibility to hypertension, irrespective of dietary factors, which characterize different genetic populations. For example, Japanese subjects exhibit a high incidence of hypertension, and autopsy studies demonstrate that this population has smaller kidneys than do Caucasians [45]. *Do these smaller kidneys contain fewer nephrons?*

Hypertension is also more common and more severe in blacks. In a study of normotensive adults, Luft et al. [46] demonstrated that, as compared to whites, black subjects had higher blood pressures with oral sodium loading, together with a decreased ability to excrete an intravenous sodium load. Helmer [47] proposed that the sensitivity of American blacks to sodium may be related to their African origins, with the tendency to retain sodium representing the consequence of the adaptation of thousands of generations to existence in tropical or subtropical conditions, with considerable stress on sodium homeostasis. Greater facility to conserve sodium, and a lesser capacity to excrete any perceived excess, could be a legacy of this geo-genetic background. While appropriate for a tropical climate, however, this ability to retain sodium would prove maladaptive in the more temperate climate of North America, thereby contributing to the high incidence of hypertension in North American blacks. Helmer [47] further suggested that this efficiency of sodium conservation might explain the predilection to low plasma renin activities in black hypertensives, a phenomenon which he was the first to identify. Black hypertensives exhibit enhanced renal vascular resistance [48], increased plasma volumes [49], and a form of hypertension which tends to respond to diuretic therapy [50], and a reduction in the glomerular capillary ultrafiltration coefficient has been postulated to contribute to this sodium retention in blacks [51]. *Could these and other low renin forms of hypertension result from a reduced number of glomeruli (or, alternatively, to a deficient filtration surface area in a normal number of glomeruli)?* By analogy, *Psammomys obesus*, the desert sand rat, has developed efficient sodium- and water-retaining ability as an adaptation to its arid environment, and values for glomerular number are higher than those in the nonadapted rat, but glomerular diameters, filtration surface areas, and single nephron glomerular filtration rates are markedly reduced [52].

Gender may also play a role in the inherited nephron number and susceptibility to hypertension. Females exhibit greater age-related increases in blood pressure than do males [34, 35] and blood pressures in black women are higher than those in black men [53]. Indeed, studies of both race and gender indicate that of all hypertensive groups, black females exhibit the greatest blood pressure increase after saline infusion, and that among normotensive subgroups, black females show the largest reductions in blood pressure following sodium and volume depletion [54]. Females have smaller kidneys than do males, and 10% fewer glomeruli [55]. *Could fewer nephrons account for these smaller kidneys and thereby contribute to enhanced susceptibility to hypertension in females?*

Nephron Number and Progression of Renal Disease

Congenital nephron endowment may also be an important determinant of the rate of progression of acquired renal disease. In the extreme case of extensive experimental renal ablation, removal of a critical portion of renal mass results in a syndrome of systemic hypertension, progressive azotemia, proteinuria, and eventual glomerular sclerosis [23, 56]. Furthermore, the pace of progression accelerates with increasing degrees of ablation. The adaptive hemodynamic response to reduced functioning nephron number is characterized by increases in the filtration rate of the remaining nephrons, the latter accomplished by increases in glomerular capillary plasma flow rate and hydraulic pressure [23, 57]. The concept that these compensatory hemodynamic changes are in fact maladaptive, contributing to ultimate glomerular destruction, is supported by observations that therapeutic interventions which limit these increases in glomerular capillary plasma flow and, especially, glomerular capillary hydraulic pressure, and effective in halting or slowing the development of chronic renal failure [23, 57–59].

Hemodynamic adaptations lead to eventual glomerular destruction not only when nephron number is reduced surgically, but also in variant rat strains born with more moderate reductions in nephron number. In the Dahl salt-sensitive rat, the 15% reduction in congenital nephron number results in single nephron hyperfiltration, hyperperfusion and glomerular capillary hypertension, with accelerated glomerular sclerosis [26, 60]. Similarly, single nephron hyperfiltration and progressive proteinuria characterize the Munich-Wistar-Fromter strain, which has fewer glomerular than its Han Wistar control [29, 30]. Though renal hemodynamics have not been studied, it seems likely that hemodynamic adaptations may also explain the relative resistance to glomerular injury that characterizes the PCG/c rat, which exhibits more glomeruli than are found in its relatively more susceptible control Wistar strain [31]. In the fawn hooded (FH) rat, which is also prone to early hypertension, proteinuria, and glomerular sclerosis, values for glomerular filtration rate and filtration fraction are higher (suggesting glomerular capillary hypertension) than in the normotensive control Wistar rat. Within the FH strain, these appears to be a subset with higher blood pressure, and accelerated development of renal injury. Glomerular numbers do no differ between the FH and Wistar rats, but have not yet been examined in the various subsets of FH rats [61]. Though nephron number is decreased in the adult Milan hypertensive rat, this strain is more resistant to development of renal injury than its normotensive control [62]. However, in contrast to the Dahl rat, the Milan hypertensive rat exhibits glomerular capillary pressures which are in fact lower than those in the normotensive strain [63], suggesting that in the established phase of hypertension at least, afferent arteriolar vasoconstriction prevents transmission of high systemic pressures to the glomerular capillary network, thus conferring relative protection from hemodynamically mediated glomerular sclerosis. In an analogous manner, while essential hypertension may result from low nephron numbers, the established phase is associated with afferent arteriolar vasoconstriction and the resulting infrequent occurrence of end-stage renal failure due solely to mild essential hypertension in humans.

Progression to end-stage renal failure is highly variable, in that rates of progression vary widely within the same disease [64, 65]. *We postulate that those individuals born with nephron numbers in the low end of the distribution curve may be the same patients who demonstrate accelerated declines in renal function following initial renal injury.* For example, a deficient congenital complement of nephrons could explain the late development of renal insufficiency in those patients who exhibit some initial recovery after acute renal failure [66], bilateral renal cortical necrosis [67], and acute post-streptococcal glomerulonephritis [68]. Conceivably, the processes of repair and compensatory hyperfiltration in surviving glomeruli could serve to preserve renal function at near-normal levels for a period of time, but the excessive hemodynamic burden imposed on a congenitally reduced filtration surface area renders this subset of patients at higher risk for eventual loss of renal function. In analogy with rat strains which exhibit decreased numbers of glomeruli, the reduced number of nephrons in such patients would bear an even greater hemodynamic burden following partial glomerular destruction by disease, exhibit even higher compensatory glomerular capillary flows and pressure, and follow an accelerated course to end-stage renal failure.

Studies in experimental animals lend support to the hypothesis that inborn nephron number may contribute to the rate of progression after renal injury. While chronic renal failure, preceded by progressive proteinuria, is the major cause of noninfectious death in laboratory rats [69], strains vary markedly in the rapidity of development of age-related renal diseases [70]. For example, Sprague-Dawley rats develop age-related proteinuria and renal lesions sooner [70], and exhibit more rapid progression to glomerular sclerosis after five-sixths nephrectomy [71] or puromycin aminonucleoside nephrosis [72], than do Munich Wistar rats. Of note, glomerular counts indicate that Sprague-Dawley rats have fewer glomeruli than do Wistar rats [73], providing a unifying explanation both for disparate rates of age-related renal injury and progression to end-stage after renal disease is acquired.

Conceivably, similar variability in congenital nephron number (i.e. filtration surface area) contributes to the observed variability in rates of decline in renal function [74] and development of glomerular sclerosis [18] seen with 'normal' human aging, as discussed above. Studies of the effects of age, race and heredity on renal function indicate that glomerular filtration rate is partially under the influence of genetic variance [54], and it seems likely that those individuals with fewer nephrons early in life are less able to maintain renal function as nephron dropout engenders hemodynamic maladaptations in remaining glomeruli. Of note, age-related loss of renal function is accelerated in North American blacks as compared to whites [53], perhaps due to a lesser number of nephrons, the legacy, as noted above, of an earlier equatorial advantage in renal salt conservation.

Inborn differences in nephron number may also contribute to susceptibility or resistance to development of renal disease in patients with diabetes mellitus. In both type I [75] and type II [76] diabetes, up to 60% of patients eventually develop diabetic glomerulopathy, while the remainder seem to be spared this complication. Those patients endowed with a reduced filtration surface might represent the subset of diabetic patients who exhibit persistent hyperfiltration early in the course of the disease, and later progression to overt diabetic glomerulopathy [77], whereas in those endowed with greater surface area, the risk of overt glomerulopathy might be less. Of note, elevated blood pressures typically precede the appearance of clinically overt diabetic glomerulopathy. Patients with type I diabetes exhibit statistical elevations in blood pressure, albeit within the normal range, when urinary albumin excretion is not yet elevated [78, 79]. During the state of incipient nephropathy, when microalbuminuria is present but prior to the development of more marked and persistent proteinuria, blood pressures are usually higher than those in normal subjects. Once diabetic glomerulopathy becomes clinically overt ($>$500 mg of albuminuria/day; serum creatinine $>$1.7 mg/dl), systemic hypertension occurs in the majority of diabetic patients [75], and severity of hypertension correlates inversely with level of renal function.

A further correlation between blood pressure and diabetes comes from the observation that those type I diabetic patients who develop renal complications are more likely to have a parent with essential hypertension [80, 81]. *Could a congenital nephron deficiency contribute to hypertension in the parent as well as to susceptibility to hypertension and glomerular injury in their diabetic offspring*?

Several other features of diabetic glomerulopathy are consistent with such a concept. Patients who develop recurrent diabetic glomerulopathy after transplantation do so in a much shorter time than was required prior to transplantation [82]; this enhanced susceptibility in the same patient may relate to the fact that the recipient has, at most, only 50% of the normal nephron number (less if the donor kidney contains fewer than one million functioning nephrons due to a congenital deficit, or nephron loss incurred during transplantation). Similarly, the relative risk of end-stage renal disease secondary to diabetic glomerulopathy is almost fourfold higher in blacks than in whites [83], perhaps again reflecting a lesser number of nephrons. Moreover, as noted above, women have smaller kidneys and fewer glomeruli than do males; black women exhibit a relative risk for diabetic glomerulopathy which is even higher than that in black males [83]. Conceivably, both race and gender contribute to a reduction in congenital filtration surface area, and enhanced risk for diabetic nephropathy.

Summary and Implications

Taken together, these experimental and clinical observations suggest that a congenital deficiency in glomerular filtration surface area contributes to two processes: limited ability to excrete sodium loads, leading to 'essential' hypertension, and susceptibility to accelerated renal failure when filtration surface area is further reduced by surgical ablation or acquired renal parenchymal disease. Reduction of nephron number, whether congenital or acquired, leads to volume-dependent systemic hypertension, and to abnormalities of neurohormonal modulators of renal excretory function including alterations in the renin-angiotensin and adrenergic nervous systems, and increased cardiac secretion of atrial natriuretic peptides. Once systemic hypertension is established, factors such as increased systemic vascular resistance and structural alterations in the renal and extrarenal vasculature tend to perpetuate the process, leading to fixed arterial hypertension. Systemic hypertension contributes to glomerular capillary hypertension, which eventuates in glomerular sclerosis. As sclerosis subsumes more and more of the glomerular filtration bed, glomerular destruction further aggravates systemic hypertension. While no therapy is yet available to directly increase inborn glomerular number or augment the growth of new glomerular capillaries, interventions which control systemic and glomerular capillary hypertension could interrupt this cycle and minimize risk in those patients most susceptible to hypertension and glomerular injury.

References

1 Ledingham JM, Cohen RD: The role of the heart in the pathogenesis of renal hypertension. Lancet 1963;ii:979.

2 Borst JGG, Borst-de Geus A: Hypertension explained by Starling's theory of circulating hemodynamics. Lancet 1963;i:677.

3 Dahl LK, Heine M, Thompson K: Genetic influence of the kidneys on blood pressure. Evidence from chronic renal homografts in rats with opposite predispositions to hypertension. Circ Res 1973;34:94.

4 Bianchi G, Fox U, DiFrancesco DF, et al: Blood pressure changes produced by kidney cross transplantation between spontaneously hypertensive rats and normotensive rats. Clin Sci Mol Med 1974;47:435.

5 Curtis JJ, Luke RG, Dustan HP, et al: Remission of essential hypertension after renal transplantation. N Engl J Med 1983;309:1009.

6 Guyton AC, Cleman PJ, Cowley AW, et al: A systems analysis approach to understanding long range arterial blood pressure control and hypertension. Circ Res 1974;35:159.

7 Fetterman GH, Habib R: Congenital bilateral oligonephronic renal hypoplasia with hypertrophy of nephrons (oligomeganephronie). Am J Clin Pathol 1969;52:199.

8 McGraw M, Poucell S, Sweet J, et al: The significance of focal segmental glomerulosclerosis in oligomeganephronia. Int J Ped Nephrol 1984;5:67.

9 Kissane JM: Congenital malformation; in Heptinstall RH (ed): Pathology of the Kidney. Boston, Little, Brown, 1966, chap 3, p 63.

10 Kiprov DD, Colvin BB, McCluskey RT: Focal and segmental glomerulosclerosis and proteinuria associated with unilateral renal agenesis. Lab Invest 1982;46:275.

11 Rugiu C, Oldrizzi L, Lupo A, et al: Clinical features of patients with solitary kidneys. Nephron 1986;43:10.

12 Thorner PS, Arbus GS, Celermajer DS, et al: Focal segmental glomerulosclerosis and progressive renal failure associated with a unilateral kidney. Pediatrics 1984;73:806.

13 Hakim R, Goldszer RC, Brenner BM: Hypertension and proteinuria: long-term sequellae of uninephrectomy in humans. Kidney Int 1984;25:930.

14 Talseth T, Fauchald P, Skrede S, et al: Long-term blood pressure and renal function in kidney donors. Kidney Int 1986;29:1072.

15 Torres VE, Offord KP, Anderson CF, et al: Blood pressure determinants in living-related allograft donors and their recipients. Kidney Int 1987;31:1383.

16 Moore RA: The total number of glomeruli in the normal human kidney. Anal Rec 1931;48:153.

17 Dunnill MS, Halley W: Some observations on the quantitative anatomy of the kidney. J Pathol 1973;110:113.

18 Kaplan C, Pasternack B, Shah H, et al: Age-related incidence of sclerotic glomeruli in human kidneys. Am J Pathol 1975;80:227.

19 Hayman JM Jr, Martin J Jr, Miller M: Renal function and the number of glomeruli in the human kidney. Arch Intern Med 1939;64:69.

20 Fetterman GH, Shuplock NA, Philipp FJ, et al: The growth and maturation of human glomeruli and proximal convolutions from term to adulthood. Studies by microdissection. Pediatrics 1965;35:601.

21 Kaysen GA, Watson JB: Mechanism of hypoalbuminemia in the 7/8-nephrectomized rat with chronic renal failure. Am J Physiol 1982;343:F372.

22 Ylitalo P, Hepp R, Oster P, et al: Effects of varying sodium intake on blood pressure and renin-angiotensin system in subtotally nephrectomized rats. J Lab Clin Med 1976;88:807.

23 Anderson S, Meyer TW, Rennke HG, et al: Control of glomerular hypertension limits glomerular injury in rats with reduced renal mass. J Clin Invest 1985;76:612.

24 Koletsky S: Role of salt and renal mass in experimental hypertension. Arch Pathol 1959;68:11.

25 Koletsky S, Goodsitt AM: Natural history and pathogenesis of renal ablation hypertension. Arch Pathol 1960;69:554.

26 Azar S, Limas C, Iwai J, et al: Single nephron dynamics during high sodium intake and early hypertension in Dahl rats. Jap Heart J 1979;20(suppl 1):138.

27 Azar S, Johnson MA, Hertel B, et al: Single-nephron pressures, flows and resistances in hypertensive kidneys with nephrosclerosis. Kidney Int 1977;12:28.

28 Baer PG, Bianchi G: Renal micropuncture study of normotensive and Milan hypertensive rats before and after development of hypertension. Kidney Int 1978;13:452.

29 Hackbarth H, Buttner D, Jarck D, et al: Distribution of glomeruli in the renal cortex of Munich Wistar Fromter (MWF) rats. Renal Physiol 1983;6:63.

30 Rovira-Halbach G, Alt JM, Brunkhorst R, et al: Single nephron hyperfiltration and proteinuria in a newly selected rat strain with superficial glomeruli. Renal Physiol 1986;9:317.

31 Grond J, Beukers JJB, Schilthuis MS, et al: Analysis of renal structural and functional features in two rat strains with a different susceptibility to glomerular sclerosis. Lab Invest 1986;54:77.

32 Azar S, Johnson MA, Scheinman J, et al: Regulation of glomerular capillary pressure and filtration rate in young Kyoto hypertensive rats. Clin Sci 1979;56:203.

33 Arendshorst WJ, Beierwaltes WH: Renal and nephron hemodynamics in spontaneously hypertensive rats. Am J Physiol 1979;236:F246.

34 Denton D: Salt intake and high blood pressure in man; in Denton D (ed): The Hunger for Salt. An Anthropological, Physiological and Medical Analysis. New York, Springer, 1982, chap 27, pp 542.

35 Page LB, Danion A, Moellering RC Jr: Antecedents of cardiovascular disease in six Solomon Islands societies. Circulation 1974;49:1132.

36 Sinnett PF, Whyte HM: Epidemiologic studies in a total highland population: Tukisenta, New Guinea. Cardiovascualr disease and relevant clinical electrocardiographic, radiologic and biochemical findings. J Chronic Dis 1973;26:265.

37 Hofman A, Hazebroek A, Valkenburg HA: A randomized trial of sodium intake and blood pressure in newborn infants. JAMA 1983;250:370.

38 Deutscher S, Epstein FH, Kjelsberg MO: Familial aggregation of factors associated with coronary heart disease. Circulation 1966;33:911.

39 Havlik RJ, Feinleib M: Epidemiology and genetics of hypertension. Hypertension 1982;4(suppl III):121.

40 Biron P, Mongeau J-G, Bertrand D: Familial aggregation of blood pressure in 558 adopted children. Can Med Ass J 1976–15:773.

41 Luft FC, Miller JZ, Weinberger MH, et al: Influence of genetic variance on sodium sensitivity of blood pressure. Klin Wochenschr 1987;65:101.

42 Grim CE, McDonough JR, Miller JZ, et al: Effects of sodium loading and depletion in normotensive first-degree relatives of essential hypertensives. J Lab Clin Med 1979;94:764.

43 Falkner B, Onesti G, Hayes P: The role of sodium in essential hypertension in genetically hypertensive adolescents; in Onesti G, Kim KE (eds): Hypertension in the Young and the Old. New York, Grune & Stratton, 1981, p 29.

44 Guidi E, Bianchi G, Rivolta E, et al: Hypertension in man with a kidney transplant: role of familial versus other factors. Nephron 1985;41:14.

45 Tauchi H, Tsuboi K, Okutomi J: Age changes in the human kidney of the different races. Gerontologia 1971;17:87.

46 Luft FC, Rankin LI, Bloch R, et al: Cardiovascular and humoral responses to extremes of sodium intake in normal black and white men. Circulation 1979;60:697.

47 Helmer OM; Hormonal and biochemical factors controlling blood pressure; Les Concepts de Claude Bernard sur le Milieu Interieur. Paris, Librairies de l'Academie de Medecine, 1967, p 115.

48 Frohlich ED, Messerli FH, Dunn FG, et al: Greater renal vascular involvement in the black patient with essential hypertension. A comparison of systemic and renal hemodynamics in black and white patients. Miner Electrolyte Metab 1984;10:173.

49 Lilley JJ, Hsu L, Stone RA: Racial disparity of plasma volume in hypertensive man. Ann Intern Med 1976;84:707.

50 Veterans Administration Cooperative Study on Antihypertensive Agents. Comparison of propranolol and hydrochlorothiazide for the initial treatment of hypertension. II. Results of long-term therapy. JAMA 1928;248:2004.

51 Luft FC, Weinberger MH, Grim CE: Sodium sensitivity and resistance in normotensive humans. Am J Med 1982;72:726.

52 Baines AD, deRouffignac C: Functional heterogeneity of nephrons. II. Filtration rates, intraluminal flow velocities and fractional water reabsorption. Pflugers Arch 1969;76:260.

53 Boyle E: Biological patterns in hypertension by race, sex, body weight and skin color. JAMA 1970;213:1637.

54 Luft FC, Fineberg NS, Miller JZ, et al: The effects of age, race and heredity on glomerular filtration rate following volume expansion and contraction in normal man. Am J Med Sci 1980;279:15.

55 McLachlan MSF, Guthrie JC, Anderson CK, et al: Vascular and glomerular changes in the aging kidney. J Pathol 1977;121:65.

56 Bourgoignie JJ, Gavellas G, Martinez E, et al: Glomerular function and morphology after renal mass reduction in dogs. J Lab Clin Med 1987;109:380.

57 Hostetter TH, Olson JL, Rennke HG, et al: Hyperfiltration in remnant nephrons: a potentially adverse response to renal ablation. Am J Physiol 1981;241:F85.

58 Brenner BM, Meyer TW, Hostetter TH: Dietary protein intake and the progressive nature of kidney disease. N Engl J Med 1982;307:652.

59 Brenner BM: Nephron adaptation to renal injury or ablation. Am J Physiol 1985;249:F324.
60 Raij L, Azar S, Keane WF: Role of hypertension in progressive glomerular immune injury. Hypertension 1985;7:398.
61 DeKeijzer MH, Provoost AP: Hyperfiltration and proteinuria in male Fawn Hooded (FH) rats with two intack kidneys developing spontaneous hypertension (Abstract). Kidney Int 1987;32:772.
62 Brandis A, Bianchi G, Realc E, et al: Age-dependent glomerulosclerosis and proteinuria occurring in rats of the Milan Normotensive Strain and not in rats of the Milan Hypertensive Strain. Lab Invest 1986;55:234.
63 Boberg U, Persson AEG: Increased tubuloglomerular feedback activity in Milan hypertensive rats. Am J Physiol 1986;250:F967.
64 Mitch WE, Walser M, Buffington GA, et al: A simple method for estimating progression of chronic renal failure. Lancet 1976;ii:1326.
65 Rutherford WE, Blondin J, Miller JP, et al: Chronic progressive renal disease: rate of change of serum creatinine concentration. Kidney Int 1977;11:62.
66 Finn WF: Recovery from acute renal failure; in Brenner BM, Lazarus JM (eds): Acute Renal Failure. Philadelphia, Saunders, 1983, chap 30, p 753.
67 Kleinknecht C, Grunfeld, Grunfeld JP, Gomez PC, et al: Diagnostic procedures and long-term prognosis in bilateral renal cortical necrosis. Kidney Int 1973;4:390.
68 Baldwin DS: Chronic glomerulonephritis: nonimmunologic mechanisms of progressive glomerular damage. Kindey Int 1982;21:109.
69 Saxton JA Jr, Kimball GC: Relation of nephrosis and other diseases of albino rats to age and to modifications of diet. Arch Pathol 1941;32:951.
70 Gray JE, van Zwieten MJ, Hollander CF: Early light microscopic changes of chronic progressive nephrosis in several strains of aging laboratory rats. J Gerontol 1982;37:142.
71 Meyer TW, Anderson S, Rennke HG, et al: Reversing glomerular hypertension stabilizes established glomerular injury. Kidney Int 1987;31:752.
72 Anderson S, Diamond JR, Karnovsky MJ, et al: Hemodynamic mechanism of glomerular sclerosis after recovery from acute nephrotic syndrome. Proc 10th Int Cong Nephrol, 1987, p 494, abstr.
73 Solomon S: Developmental changes in nephron number, proximal tubular length and superficial nephron glomerular filtration rate of rats. J Physiol 1977;272:573.
74 Davies DF, Shock NW: Age changes in glomerular filtration rate, effective renal plasma flow, and tubular excretory capacity in adult males. J Clin Invest 1950;29:496.
75 Hasslacher C, Ritz E, Terpstra J, et al: Natural history of nephrology in type I diabetes. Relationship to metabolic control and blood pressure. Hypertension 1985;7(suppl II):74.
76 Hasslacher C, Wahl P, Ritz E: Similar risks of nephropathy in type I and type II diabetes (Abstract). Kidney Int 1988;33:193.
77 Mogensen CE, Christensen CK: Predicting diabetic nephropathy in insulin-dependent patients. N Engl J Med 1984;311:89.
78 Feldt-Rasmussen B, Borch-Johnsen K, Mathiesen ER: Hypertension in diabetes as related to nephropathy. Early blood pressure changes. Hypertension 1985;7(suppl II):18.
79 Mogensen CE, Christensen CK: Blood pressure changes and renal function in incipient and overt diabetic nephropathy. Hypertension 1985;7(suppl II):64.
80 Krolewski AS, Canessa M, Rand LI, et al: Genetic predisposition to hypertension as a major determinant of development of diabetic nephropathy (Abstract). Kidney Int 1987;31:388A.
81 Viberti GC: ACE inhibition and the diabetic kidney. R Soc Med Round Table Series, in press.

82 Mauer SM, Steffes MW, Connett J, et al: The development of lesions in the glomerular basement membrane and mesangium after transplantation of normal kidneys to diabetic patients. Diabetes 1983;32:948.
83 Kappal DF, Van Tuinen M: Trends in the incidence of treated end-stage renal disease secondary to diabetic nephropathy. Am J Kidney Dis 1986;8:234.

Barry M. Brenner, MD, Renal Division, Brigham and Women's Hospital,
75 Francis Street, Boston, MA 02115 (USA)

Oldrizzi L, Maschio G, Rugiu C, et al. (eds): The Progressive Nature of Renal Disease: Myths and Facts. Contrib Nephrol. Basel, Karger, 1989, vol 75, pp 60–67

Is Chronic Renal Disease Always Progressive?

Jonas Bergström, Anders Alvestrand, Härje Bucht, Alberto Gutierrez, Peter Stenvinkel

Department of Renal Medicine, Karolinska Institute, Huddinge University Hospital, Stockholm, Sweden

It is a common experience that chronic renal disease with reduction in renal function exorably progresses to end-stage renal failure. However, the progression rate varies widely between different patients which may be attributed to several factors such as the underlying renal disease, the activity of the disease process, hypertension, proteinuria and dietary and metabolic factors. In the last few years the possibility to retard or forestall the progression of renal failure has been explored both in animal models and in patients [1]. Various groups have presented data which suggest that the progression may be retarded by treatment with a low protein intake. Control of hypertension also seems to influence the progression of renal failure.

In this communication, results from two studies performed in Stockholm will be briefly summarized. One study is a retrospective survey of factors associated with progression in patients with early renal failure. The other is a prospective study of low-protein diet on the progression of chronic renal failure, the Stockholm Prospective Randomized Study, which is still going on.

Retrospective Study of the Progression Rate of Renal Failure in Various Diseases

Material and Methods

We reviewed the medical records of all non-diabetic patients with chronic renal disease with a serum creatinine concentration (s-Cr) of 200–350 μmol/l attending the out-patients clinic of the Department of Renal Medicine at Huddinge University Hospital between October 6, 1980, and December 31, 1986, in whom it was possible to assess the rate of progression of renal failure (i.e. patients in whom at least four s-Cr determinations had been made over a period of 6 months or longer after an initial determination of a s-Cr of 200–350 μmol/l.

In each patient the average value of all records of blood pressure (measured after 5–10 min of rest in the supine position) over the observation period was calculated. Several

Table 1. Mean arterial pressure (MAP) and urinary protein excretion (UPE) in the four diagnosis groups of the retrospective study (mean $\pm$ SD)

	n	MAP, mm Hg	UPE, g/24 h
Chronic glomerulonephritis	29	110 ± 8	5.4 ± 3.3
Chronic interstitial nephritis	24	105 ± 10	1.8 ± 1.6
Polycystic kidney disease	20	109 ± 9	1.4 ± 1.2
Mixed group	26	112 ± 10	3.2 ± 2.9

patients took antihypertensive drugs, including diuretics, β-blocking agents, calcium channel blockers, ACE inhibitors and vasodilatory drugs. For each patient the number of hypertensive drugs taken simultaneously was averaged over the observation period. The average urinary protein excretion (UPI) was calculated from determinations of protein in 24-hour urine samples, collected over the observation period.

The rate of progression of renal failure was evaluated from the linear regression of the reciprocal of s-Cr (mmol/l) on time (months), and the regression coefficient (b) was used as an index of the progression rate. Using arbitrarily chosen limits for b we divided the cases into three different groups of progression: Group FP (fast progression), $b < -0.05$; group SP (slow progression), $-0.01 > b > -0.05$; group NP (no progression), $b > -0.01$. In the final evaluation patients showing no progression with a shorter observation period than 48 months were excluded.

Patients Material

Of 126 patients, 18 in group NP were excluded from the final evaluation because of a too short observation time (<48 months). Of the remaining 108 patients 38 had a medical history suggesting chronic glomerulonephritis (CGN), confirmed by renal biopsy in 29 cases. 24 patients had chronic interstitial nephritis (CIN) (14 pyelonephritis) diagnosed on basis of i.v. urogram, postmortem examinations or a history of reflux. Twenty patients had polycystic kidney disease (PCK). The remaining 26 patients (mixed group) was heterogenous with regard to diagnoses. The observation period ranged from 8 to 63 months, mean 30 ± 15 months. No patient was treated with low-protein diet over the observation period except for symptomatic treatment of near end-stage renal failure.

Table 1 shows the mean blood pressure and urinary protein excretion in the four diagnosis groups. MAP was approximately equal in all groups while UPE was on average higher in the patients with CGN and in the mixed group.

Seventeen patients (16%) showed no progression (s-Cr: initial 251 ± 35, final 221 ± 244 μmol/l; observation time 54 ± 4 months). Thirty-two (30%) had slow progression (s-Cr initial 253 ± 46, final 508 ± 340 μmol/l; observation time 46 ± 12 months) and 59 patients (55%) had fast progression (s-Cr initial 235 ± 34, final 744 ± 314 μmol/l; observation time 29 ± 13 months).

Figure 1 shows the rate of progression in patients with CGN, CIN and PCK. The figure demonstrates that the majority of patients with CGN (66%) had fast progression whereas only one was in the no-progression group. Patients with CIN were equally distributed between the three groups of progression. The majority of patients with PCK (75%) had fast progression and none of these patients had no progression. In the mixed group 8 of 17 patients (47%) had no progression.

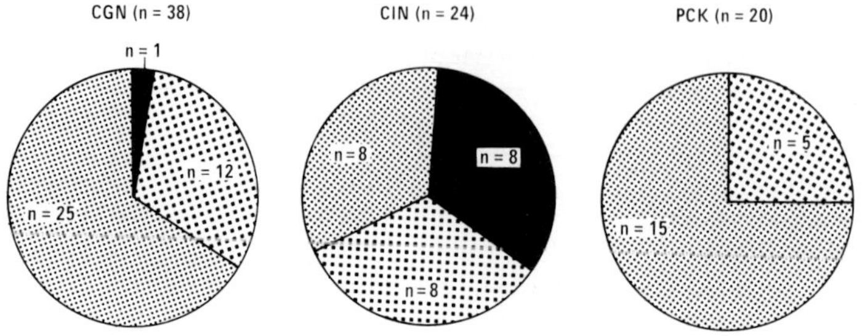

Fig. 1. Progression rates within the diagnostic groups. NP = No progression (black areas); SP = slow progression (cross-hatched areas); FP = fast progression (grey areas); CGN = chronic glomerulonephritis; CIN = chronic interstitial nephritis; PCK = polycystic kidney disease.

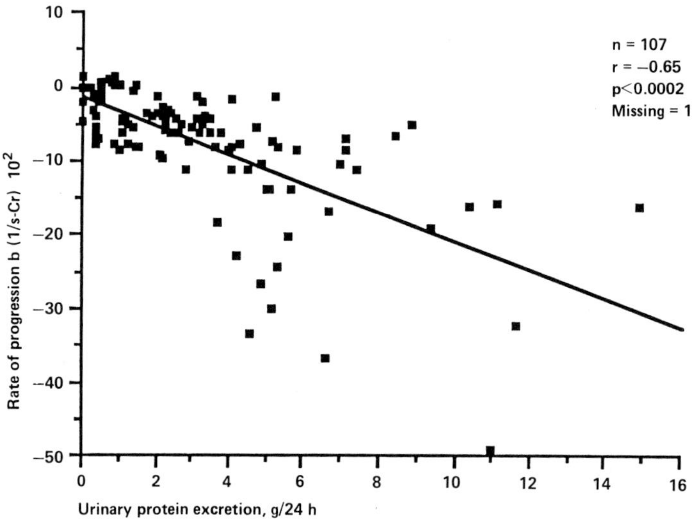

Fig. 2. Correlation of rate of progression and urinary protein excretion in the retrospective study. A more negative b-value means fast progression.

The urinary protein excretion was correlated to the progression rate in the whole material (fig. 2) and also in the subgroups with CGN, CIN and PCK.

In the total material the patients with no progression (group NP) had significantly lower MAP (103 ± 8) than group SP (110 ± 9; $p < 0.05$) and FP (111 ± 9; $p < 0.01$). In group NP the average number of antihypertensive drugs taken simultaneously (mean 1.2) was significantly lower than in group SP (mean 1.9; $p < 0.01$) and FP (mean 2.1; $p < 0.001$).

Comment

The results of this study show that the mean progression rate varies with the diagnosis but also demonstrates that the progression rate may vary considerably within each diagnosis group. No less than 16% of all patients had no progression according to our criteria; practically all these patients belonged to the CIN or mixed diagnosis group. On the other hand a majority of the patients with CGN and PCK showed fast progression, the mean rate of progression being highest in the CGN group. The findings of relatively rapid progression in PCK was unexpected since it is generally believed that the progression of renal failure is slow in this disease.

In the total material patients with progression (group SP and FP) both had higher blood pressure than the patients with no progression who also required less antihypertensive therapy, indicating that hypertension is an important factor for progression of renal failure in man. Finally, the rate of progression was correlated with UPI irrespective of diagnosis. The association between proteinuria and rate of progression suggests that excessive glomerular filtration of protein may be a factor which promotes the development of glomerulosclerosis, but may also reflect a higher activity of the underlying disease process.

The Stockholm Prospective Randomized Study

Design of the Study

The purpose of this study was originally to assess the effect of protein restriction on the progression of chronic renal failure. The study was started in June 1983 and is still going on. Included in the study are patients with creatinine clearance <70 ml/min/1.73 m^2 and approximately linear progression of renal failure, who volunteered to participate. Patients with systemic disease (diabetes, SLE, etc.), nephrotic syndrome (UPI ≥ 6 g/24 h) and patients treated with corticosteroids, immunosuppressive drugs and non-steroid anti-inflammatory drugs are excluded. Before being randomized into two groups, one with uncontrolled protein intake and one with low-protein diet, the patients enter a prospective control phase for 12 months and, in the case of no significant progression over this period, for another 12 months. Only patients who show evidence of progression after 12 or 24 months, respectively, are then randomized. Criteria for progression evaluated from the correlation between reciprocal of s-Cr and time (significance of the correlation coefficient, r) were as follows: During 24 months: $t \geq 2.306$, $p \leq 0.05$, 10 or more determinations; during 24 months: $t \geq 2.101$, $p \leq 0.05$, $n = 20$. During the prospective control phase and after randomization the patients are seen in the same centre, by the same physicians and other staff members with the same frequency. Blood pressure, blood chemistry, 24-hour creatinine clearances and 24-hour UPI are determined every month as are s-Cr and ^{51}Cr-EDTA clearance. Our aim is to keep the blood pressure below 160/90, plasma bicarbonate ≥ 20 mmol/l and serum phosphate ≤ 1.7 mmol/l. Clinical and laboratory checkups (once per month) were considerably more frequent during the prospective control phase than during the previous retrospective phase.

When we compared progression during the retrospective and prospective phase, the 24-hour creatinine clearance and the reciprocal of s-Cr, respectively, on time were calculated and the regression coefficients (b-values) used as indices of the progression rate. ^{51}Cr-EDTA clearance could not be used since repeated determinations were not available during the retrospective phase in most patients.

When we analysed our first 17 patients we found that the progression rate decreased significantly after the patients entered the prospective control phase, i.e. without changing the dietary intake of protein and that the degree of retardation was correlated to improved blood pressure control [2]. Since then an increasing number of patients have been accepted for the study and in the following we will give a report on the outcome based on a larger material of patients.

Progress Report

Until now (September 1988) 57 cases have entered the prospective study, of which 13 cases are still in the control phase and cannot be evaluated with regard to progression; 3 cases have withdrawn. Of the remaining 41 patients 23 progressed during the control phase and were randomized and 8 progressed to end-stage renal failure. However, in no less than 10 patients (24%) no progression at all (according to our criteria) was noticed over the prospective study period of more than 2 years (on non-restricted protein intake), and in several of the other patients the rate of progression decreased significantly during the prospective period in comparision to the retrospective period.

A closer analysis was made in 28 patients in whom repeated determinations of serum-creatinine and creatinine clearance were available retrospectively (mean 579, range 125–740 days) as well as prospectively (mean 493, range 216–742 days [3]. The patient material is characterized in table 2. In 17 of the patients the rate of progression decreased significantly whereas in 8 patients the rate increased after entering the prospective phase.

There was a strongly significant correlation between the change in mean arterial pressure (ΔMAP) and the change in progression rate comparing the retrospective to the prospective period. Both evaluated from the reciprocal of s-Cr ($r = 0.48$, $n = 28$; $p < 0.01$) and from the creatinine

Table 2. Data from 28 patients with chronic renal failure before entering the prospective, randomized study (mean ± SD)

Diagnosis	n	Blood pressure mm Hg		Creatinine clearance ml/min	Urinary protein excretion ml/24 h
		systolic	diastolic		
CGN	12	149 ± 18	93 ± 3	38 ± 14	2.7 ± 1.7
CIN	7	136 ± 8	89 ± 7	25 ± 4	3.5 ± 1.4
PCK	8	143 ± 9	92 ± 4	23 ± 9	2.7 ± 1.9
Nephrosclerosis	1	113	84	31	3.5

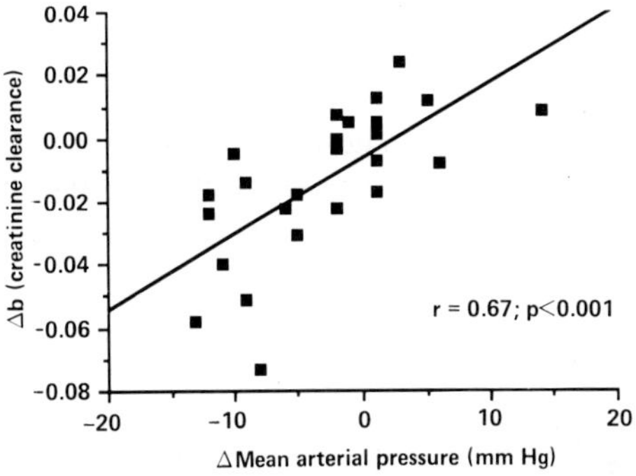

Fig. 3. Correlation between changes (prospective-retrospective phase) in mean arterial pressure and changes in progression of renal failure (changes in regression coefficient of creatinine clearance, ml/min on time, days). A negative value of b indicates retardation of progression [from ref. 3, with the permission of the editor] (n = 25).

clearance (fig. 3). The correlation between ΔMAP and Δ creatinine clearance was significant for the patients with CGN ($r = 0.74$, $n = 12$; $p < 0.01$); in the patients with CIN and PCK the r-values were high ($r = 0.83$, $n = 5$ and $r = 0.70$, $n = 7$; respectively) although not attaining statistical significance ($p < 0.1$) because of the small number of patients in each group.

In figure 4 the progression rate of renal failure during the retrospective and prospective periods have been plotted against the mean blood pressure for each case. The figure demonstrates that a fall in mean blood pressure is associated with a decrease in progression rate and that the effect of blood pressure reduction appears to be larger at higher blood pressure levels. The association was however also apparent at mean blood pressure levels as low as 100–110 mm Hg.

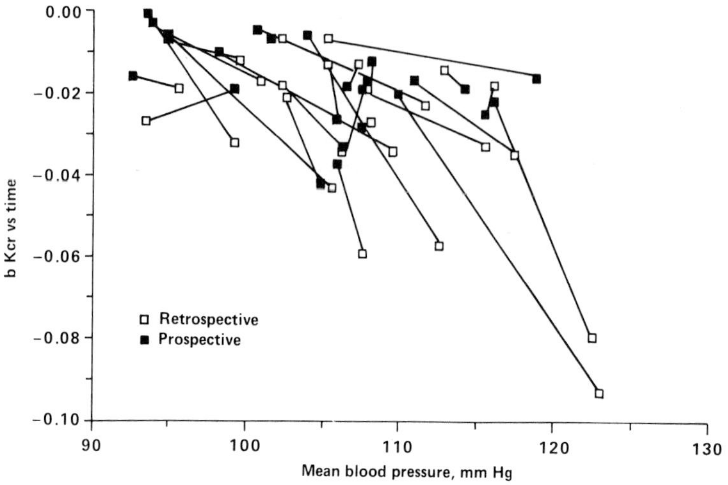

Fig. 4. Mean blood pressure and mean progression rate, i.e. the regression coefficient of creatinine clearance, ml/min, on time, days (b Kcr vs time) during the retrospective and prospective phase.

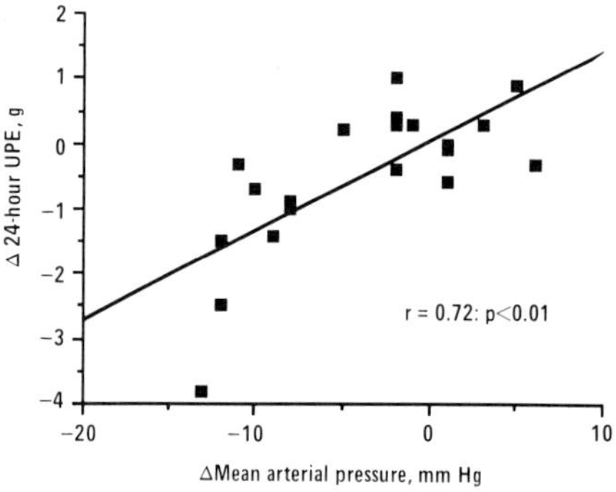

Fig. 5. Correlation between changes (retrospective-prospective phase) in mean arterial pressure and changes in 24-hour protein excretion in whom protein excretion was quantified both in the retrospective and prospective phase [from ref. 3, with the permission of the editor].

For all patients in whom protein excretion was measured in both study periods a significant correlation ($p < 0.001$) was found between change in mean blood pressure and urinary protein excretion (fig. 5). This correlation reached statistical significance ($p < 0.01$) also in patients with chronic glomerulonephritis.

Comment

The results of this study corroborates the finding of the retrospective study that chronic renal failure is not always progressive. Moreover, it indicates that progression can be retarded or even halted completely by more proper medical care with better control of hypertension pressure. The results suggest that mild hypertension or even 'high' normal blood pressure, i.e. in the range of 140–180–150/90 should be treated and that the goal should be to keep the patient at a blood pressure level around 120–130/80 rather than 150/90 in order to prevent progression. Better blood pressure control was also associated with lower protein excretion, suggesting that reduction of systemic blood pressure has a beneficial effect on intra-glomerular haemodynamics.

In our study most patients were treated with various combinations of diuretic, vasodilatory and β-blocking agents. Whether ACE-blocking drugs afford any advantage over conventional antihypertensive therapy in man with regard to prevention of progression of renal failure is still an open question and would require prospective controlled studies for an answer.

References

1 Klahr S, Schreiner G, Ichikawa I: The progression of renal disease. N Engl J Med 1988;318:1657–1666.

2 Bergström J, Alvestrand A, Bucht H, Gutierrez A: Progression of chronic renal failure in man is retarded with more frequent clinical follow-ups and better blood pressure control. Clin Nephrol 1986;25:1–6.

3 Alvestrand A, Gutierrez A, Bucht H, Bergström J: Reduction of blood pressure retards the progression of chronic renal failure in man. Nephrol Dial Transplant 1988, in press.

Prof. Jonas Bergström, Department of Renal Medicine, Huddinge University Hospital, S-141 86 Huddinge (Sweden)

Oldrizzi L, Maschio G, Rugiu C, et al. (eds): The Progressive Nature of Renal Disease: Myths and Facts. Contrib Nephrol. Basel, Karger, 1989, vol 75, pp 68–75

The Natural History of Glomerulonephritis

J. Stewart Cameron

Renal Unit, Department of Medicine, Guy's Campus, UMDS, London, England, UK

I have written twice in the past on this subject in some detail [1, 2] and the reader is referred to these two articles for the literature on the subject up to 1985.

Clinical Factors Associated with Differences in Prognosis in Glomerulonephritis

Age

A child's kidney is likely to be able to recover more completely and quickly than an adult's, since the child's kidney is still growing in size and function. Similarly the elderly might suffer a poorer prognosis than that observed in younger adults. Finally in Western societies at least, blood pressures rise with age in healthy populations. Tables 1 and 2 summarize data from the literature on the long-term outcome of various forms of glomerular disease at various ages.

In *focal segmental sclerosis/hyalinosis* (FSGS) there is a lower proportion of adults who enter complete remission on initial courses of prednisolone in conventional dosage [3]. In children and adolescents, a particularly vicious form of disease is seen which is absent in adults: so-called 'malignant FSGS', often with immediate or early recurrence of proteinuria and then sclerosing lesions in renal allografts.

In *IgA-associated nephropathy*, there are surprisingly few data from long-term follow-up of children to compare with the wealth of data from adults. More children than adults present with macroscopic haematuria, have little or no associated proteinuria, and few develop chronic renal failure.

In the *vasculitides* it is almost impossible to make comparisons, since Henoch-Schönlein purpura is so overwhelmingly a disease of the young, whilst *microscopic polyarteritis* and *Wegener's granuloma* are so much diseases of the middle-aged and elderly, but in adults we [4] showed that vasculitic patients aged over 60 did worse than younger patients.

Table 1. Effect of age on outcome in non-proliferative glomerulopathies

Minimal change disease	gradient of age in frequency of relapses – young children <adults < elderly children more frequently respond to steroids (94 vs 75–85%) ?children more rapidly respond to steroids children more rapidly respond to cyclophosphamide
Focal segmental glomerulosclerosis	children more frequently respond to steroids (29 vs 19%) children less often enter renal failure
Membranous nephropathy	children rarely go into renal failure older adults do worse than younger (or the same) according to author

There are good data that children with *lupus* more frequently show overt clinical nephritis [5], whilst those with an onset over 50 years of age show this less frequently than young adults [6]. Equally lupus nephritis in prepubertal children is more often severe, resistant to treatment and fatal, whilst the rather rare lupus nephritis in the middle-aged and elderly is often mild, and runs a benign course, at least under treatment [6]. However some adult series show no effect of age on outcome.

Sex

The majority of glomerulonephritides affect males more than females; the notable exceptions are of course lupus, and mesangiocapillary glomerulonephritis.

In *membranous nephropathy* and *IgA-associated nephropathy* males do worse than females. In *mesangiocapillary nephritis*, however, the situation is not so clear: Magil et al. [7] reported a worse outcome for males, but most series have found no difference between the sexes. No comment is made in the literature on sex as a factor in *acute endocapillary glomerulonephritis*, or in *vasculitis*, although in one series boys with HSP nephritis were reported to do worse than females.

One can only speculate why males should in general do worse than females in glomerular diseases. Males not only do not live as long as females even when healthy, but also have, age for age, higher blood pressures in Western societies from which our data are drawn.

Whether maleness per se, e.g. some hormonal effect, is at work directly on the kidney is unknown. Differences in protein or salt intake between the

Table 2. Effect of age on outcome in proliferative glomerulopathies

Acute endocapillary nephritis	young children almost never progress older children rarely progress adults more frequently progress ? elderly often progress
Mesangiocapillary glomerulonephritis	? children do better than adults
Dense deposit disease	? children do better than adults
IgA-associated nephropathy	children rarely go into renal failure adults sometimes go into renal failure elderly do worse
Crescentic glomerulonephritis	? no difference with age
Microscopic vasculitis	uncommon in children; elderly do worse
HSP nephritis	older children do worse than younger adults do about as well as children
Lupus nephritis	children probably higher incidence of nephritis probably do worse than adults middle-aged and elderly: less often nephritis milder disease

sexes, or an indirect effect of sex hormones on their handling, are other possibilities to be considered.

Obviously *lupus* is a special case since there is good animal evidence that the sexual phenotype and oestrogen levels have a powerful influence on the appearance of the disease. However, in those few males affected by lupus, the appearance of clinical nephritis is as common (ca 45%) as in females, and in males the nephritis appears to run an approximately parallel course [8].

Race

There are few data which suggest that the race Caucasian, oriental or black has an influence on the outcome of any form of primary glomerular disease, although there are striking differences in the incidence of different types of nephritis in different countries, even in the West. It has been suggested, but also denied, that lupus nephritis is more frequently severe in orientals and blacks than in Caucasians.

MHC Type

A number of relatively weak, and two strong associations with MHC types have been described in glomerulopathies [9]. The strong associations are between anti-GBM nephritis and HLA-DR2, and membranous nephropathy and HLA-DR3, at least in European Caucasians; in Japan, the association is with HLA-DR2.

It has been suggested that in both anti-GBM disease and in membranous nephropathy the strong DR association interacts with other MHC antigens to give a higher risk for progression. In *anti-GBM nephritis*, an association of DR2 with B7 was accompanied by a more severe onset and poorer outlook for renal function [10]; no confirmatory study has been done. In *membranous nephropathy*, association of DR3 with B8 and BfF1 seemed to show a somewhat poorer prognosis [11] but this was not confirmed in a more recent larger study of the British Medical Research Council (MRC) trial of prednisolone in membranous nephropathy.

Finally, an extended MHC haplotype was described in association with *mesangiocapillary glomerulonephritis* types I and III: B8-DR3-SC01-GL02 associated also with a poorer outlook for renal function [12]. No confirmatory studies have yet been done.

Hypertension

This topic was discussed in detail in a previous Verona symposium, which volume should be consulted [13]. Almost all authors agree that in almost all chronic glomerulopathies the presence of raised blood pressure or the requirement for hypotensive treatment is associated with a poorer outlook for renal function, and often for the whole patient. Further, the superimposition of diastolic hypertension on experimental models of glomerulopathy is well known to accelerate renal damage.

The exception to this rule is of course those conditions in which an acute nephritic onset, accompanied by even severe hypertension, is a feature of the disease. Thus the *initial* blood pressure is a poor prognostic indictor in mesangiocapillary glomerulonephritis, and an irrelevant finding for outcome in acute endocapillary glomerulonephritis and Henoch-Schönlein purpura.

In addition, in vasculitis and in anti-GBM nephritis – indeed all forms of crescentic glomerulonephritis where glomerular tuft necrosis rather than proliferation/infiltration is present – hypertension is rare, volume-dependent, usually mild, and irrelevant to prognosis. Possible mechanisms of acceleration of renal damage by hypertension are discussed in reference [13].

Proteinuria

The relationship between the presence and/or the degree of proteinuria and prognosis is an interesting one. Obviously, looking at glomerular diseases globally the presence of profuse proteinuria is *not* a prognostic feature, since those patients who do best with regard to long-term renal function – those with *minimal change disease* – are amongst those with the greatest proteinuria.

However, if we look at the degree of proteinuria in those patients with a predominantly haematuric presentation, or with chronic disease, a striking association of outcome with presence and degree of proteinuria emerges [1, 14]. In IgA-associated nephropathy, every series has reported that those patients who do badly have proteinuria as well as haematuria, and that in those entering terminal renal failure eventually, it may be several grams per day or of nephrotic dimensions [15].

In the three classic primary chronic proteinuric glomerulonephritides – *mesangiocapillary nephritis*, *membranous nephropathy* and *FSGS* – patients with proteinuria of nephrotic dimensions at presentation do worse than those with lesser degrees of proteinuria. In all three appearances, as well as in IgA nephropathy, more that 2 g/24 h proteinuria persisting in all specimens taken beyond the first 2 or 3 years of follow-up is a marker for eventual renal failure in the majority [1]. A few patients in this group, however, preserve normal renal function (see below) and go into late remission.

In *lupus nephritis*, the situation is made more encouraging but also more difficult to interpret by the fact that treatment will reliably affect proteinuria. Thus most series of treated patients do not report an association between a nephrotic syndrome at onset and outcome, although a few sets of data do. Presumably this reflects more of the 'natural' untreated outcome of the disease.

This strong association between persisting proteinuria and poor outcome in patients with structurally damaged glomeruli provokes speculation. Is the proteinuria merely a marker for more severe glomerular damage, of activity of whatever process may be going on in the glomeruli, such as glomerular capillary hypertension? Or is proteinuria in some way of itself intrinsically damaging? At the moment we cannot decide, but two possibilities by which profuse proteinuria itself might be damaging come to mind.

The first is that the chronic transit of large amounts of protein across glomerular capillary basement membranes, and through the mesangium and/or epithelial cells damages these structures [16]. Proteinuria occurs in remnant kidney rats, and even in corticosteroid-responsive relapsing nephrotic syndrome in man, global and segmental scerosis of up to half the glomeruli may be evident after 10 years or more of even intermittent proteinuria. Experimentally, the injection of large amounts of heterologous protein leads to 'overflow' heterologous proteinuria, but then leads to persistent autologous proteinuria and progressive epithelial cell damage.

The second possibility is that the alterations in coagulation mechanisms brought about by the proteinuria, and in particular the platelet hyperaggregability, may lead to intraglomerular thrombosis, inflammation and damage as in remnant kidneys [16]. These two suggestions are not of course mutually exclusive; both might operate.

Renal Function

Renal function at presentation is a *surprisingly poor indicator* of outcome unless the histology of the glomeruli is taken into account. In *acute endocapillary glomerulonephritis* a major degree of uraemia, or a requirement for dialysis may be present with subsequent complete recovery. The same is true of *Henoch-Schönlein purpura*. In *crescentic* forms of glomerulonephritis, however, the prognosis *is* significantly related to the degree of renal function, especially in relation to the start of treatment. Thus, in both *vasculitis* and *anti-GBM disease*, the outlook for renal function is better if renal function is still preserved when the patient arrives for investigation and treatment. Even with treatment by plasma exchange and cyclophosphamide, in anti-GBM disease recovery of renal function after requirement for dialysis is distinctly rare [17].

In chronic proteinuric or nephrotic types of glomerulopathy even *minimal change* in renal function may be depressed at onset without structural damage being present. Information on initial renal function within groups such as *membranous nephropathy*, however, is useful in distinguishing those who do badly, although the discrimination is poor; plasma creatinines at onset predicted those at 3 years in the nephrotic patients with membranous nephropathy in the British MCR trial.

The main value of measurements of renal function in proteinuric patients for prognosis lies, however, in *serial measurements* in those with persisting proteinuria [1]. After only 2–3 years, the great majority of those who will eventually develop renal failure will have raised plasma creatinine concentrations ($>130\ \mu$mol/l), and no doubt formal GFR measurements would pick this group out even earlier. Conversely the maintenance of normal stable or near normal function for only 2–3 years is a very encouraging sign, even though a full nephrotic syndrome may be causing worry.

Histological Features Associated with Decline in Renal Function

Tubulointerstitial Lesions

The striking, central feature is that it is not changes in the glomeruli which best predict renal function and outcome, but the severity and extent of changes in the *tubules and interstitium* [18]. This seems to be true of IgA nephropathy, focal segmental sclerosis, membranous nephropathy, mesangiocapillary nephritis, lupus nephritis, and even crescentic nephritis to some extent. This suggests that tubulointerstitial events may be crucial in determining prognosis [18].

Glomerular Lesions

In *crescentic nephritis*, however, some good pointers to prognosis can be found within or around the glomeruli: obvious intraglomerular proliferation (relatively good) of immune deposits of immunoglobulins or 'humps' visible on electron microscopy (relatively good) and the extent of crescent formation (bad with increasing involvement, especially if Bowman's capsule is ruptured). 'Good' and 'bad' in the context of this group of course relate to a general poor prognosis in comparison to almost every other group studied.

Overall, glomerulosclerosis might be expected to be a good indicator of function and prognosis, but in practice is much poorer than expected, and certainly worse than tubular sclerosis. In *IgA nephropathy*, however, the presence of segmental glomerulosclerosis is a reliable indicator of poor prognosis, perhaps because in this appearance it is usually absent.

In *membranous nephropathy*, the so-called staging of the changes into grades I–IV relates poorly or not at all to outcome in different series. In *focal segmental glomerulosclerosis* it has been alleged that the site of the lesion within the glomeruli predicts outcome [19], peri-hilar lesions being bad in this respect, and peripheral or 'tip' lesions good. This suggestion does not appear to be holding up under further examination [Chaudhury et al., in preparation; White, personal communication].

In *lupus nephritis*, as well as the tubulointerstitial changes being valuable, the appearance of the glomeruli also gives useful information. This relates not so much to the appearances classified into WHO grades I–IV and V, but the amount of glomerulosclerosis on the one hand ('chronicity') and the changes of 'activity' on the other (capillary thrombi, nuclear dusting, necrotic lesions, etc.). Similarly in *Henoch-Schönlein purpura* nephritis, apart from the frequency and periglomerular extent of any crescents, the amount of mesangial expansion associates with chronicity or decline in renal function.

Conclusions

Many factors can be identified which associate with a good or bad prognosis in glomerulonephritic patients. Most of these appear to be to some extent additive, so that whilst exceptions abound, the archetype of a patient with a poor prognosis is an older, hypertensive nephrotic male with extensive tubular atrophy, interstitial fibrosis and glomerulosclerosis, already with diminished renal function; whilst in contrast the ideal patient with a good prognosis is a young normotensive modestly proteinuric female, without any renal scarring on biopsy.

References

1 Cameron JS: The natural history of nephritis; in Black DAK, Jones NF (eds): Renal Disease. Oxford, Blackwell, 1979, pp 329–382.
2 Cameron JS: The long-term outcome of glomerular diseases; in Schrier RW, Gottschalk, CW (eds): Strauss and Welt's Diseases of the Kidney; ed 4. Boston, Little, Brown, 1988, pp 2127–2189.
3 Schena P, Cameron JS: The treatment of proteinuric idiopathic glomerulonephritis in adults: a retrospective survey. Am J Med 1988 (in press).
4 Serra A, Cameron JS: Renal vasculitis in the aged; in Nunez JM, Cameron JS (eds): Renal Function and Disease in the Elderly. London, Butterworth, 1987, pp 321–347.
5 Cameron JS: Lupus nephritis in childhood; in Edelmann CE, Spitzer A, Travis LB, Meadow SR (eds): Pediatric Kidney Disease. Boston, Little, Brown, 1989.
6 Wilson HA, Hamilton ME, Spyker DA, et al: Age influences the clinical and serologic expression of systemic lupus erythematosus. Arthritis Rheum 1981;24:1230–1235.
7 Magil AB, Price JDE, Bower S, et al: Membranoproliferative glomerulonephritis type 1: comparison of natural history in children and adults. Clin Nephrol 1979;11:239–244.
8 Miller MH, Urowitz MB, Gladman DD, et al: Systemic lupus erythematosus in males. Medicine 1983;62:327–334.
9 Rees AJ: The HLA complex and susceptibility to glomerulonephritis. Plasma Ther Transfus Technol 1984;5:455–470.
10 Rees AJ, Peters DK, Amos N, et al: The influence of HLA-linked genes on the severity of anti-GBM antibody-mediated nephritis. Kidney Int 1984;26:444–450.
11 Short CD, Dyer PA, Cairns SA, et al: A major histocompatibility system haplotype associated with poor prognosis in idiopathic membranous nephropathy. Dis Markers 1983;1:189–196.
12 Welch TR, Beischel L, Balakrishnan K, et al: Major histocompatibility complex extended haplotypes in membranoproliferative glomerulonephritis. N Engl J Med 1986;314:1476–1481.
13 Maschio G, Campese VM, Valvo E, et al: Hypertension and renal disease. Contr Nephol 1986;54:1–230.
14 Williams PS, Fass G, Bone JM: Renal pathology and proteinuria determine progression in untreated mild/moderate chronic renal failure. Q J Med 1988;67:343–354.
15 D'Amico G, Minetti L, Ponticelli C, et al: Prognostic indicators in idopathic IgA mesangial nephropathy. Q J Med 1986;59:363–378.
16 Klahr S, Schreiner G, Ichikawa I: Progression in renal disease. N Engl J Med 1988;318:1657–1666.
17 Rees AJ, Lockwood CM: Antiglomerular basement membrane antibody-mediated nephritis; in Schrier RW, Gottschalk CW (eds): Strauss and Welt's Diseases of the Kidney; ed 4. Boston, Little, Brown, 1988, pp 2091–2126.
18 Cameron JS: Immunologically mediated interstitial nephritis: tubulointerstitial nephritis: primary and secondary. Adv Nephrol 1988;18.
19 Ito H, Yoshikawa N, Aozai F, et al: Twenty-seven children with focal segmental glomerulosclerosis: correlation between the segmental location of the glomerular lesions and prognosis. Clin Nephrol 1984;22:9–14.

Prof. J.S. Cameron, Clinical Science Labs, 17th Floor, Guy's Tower,
Guy's Hospital, London SE1 9RT (UK)

Oldrizzi L, Maschio G, Rugiu C, et al. (eds): The Progressive Nature of Renal Disease: Myths and Facts. Contrib Nephrol. Basel, Karger, 1989, vol 75, pp 76–81

Factors of Progression in IgA Mesangial Nephropathy

G. D'Amico, A. Ragni, R. Torpia

Division of Nephrology, S. Carlo Hospital, Milano, Italia

It is not known yet what the mechanisms of progression of chronic glomerulonephritides (GN) are. Even more, we do not know yet if relentless progression always occurs in such diseases. In the last few years, we have been trying to answer these questions, in our study of the natural history of a large number of patients with a single type of chronic primary GN, idiopathic IgA mesangial nephropathy [1, 2], which is presumably die to the damaging effect of the long-lasting mesangial (and sometimes also parietal) deposition of circulating IgA-immune complexes or IgA antibodies [3–5].

For the following reasons this disease appears to be a good model: (1) It always has a chronic course (there has never been described, to our knowledge, a spontaneous disappearance of mesangial deposits at immunofluorescence (IF) or the regression of the glomerular lesions, that have been documented by a previous biopsy, even though there can be prolonged disappearance of all the clinical signs of activity of the disease in a minority of patients). (2) The rate of progression to end-stage renal failure (ESRF) in the various patients is quite variable (in other words, the mechanisms responsible for the progression cause a variable damage in different patients, providing better insight into their nature and their interrelationship with the patient-related, possibly genetic, factors that induce variable responses to the same damaging mechanisms). (3) The majority of patients with this disease are not treated at all throughout the entire course of the disease (and, therefore, there is not interference from therapeutic factors with the spontaneous course of the disease).

We have analyzed the various histological and clinical risk-factors in a large population of adult patients with idiopathic IgA mesangial nephropathy, with a mean follow-up from the apparent onset now longer than 10 years, and for whom the calculated renal survival has been 93% at 5 years, 85.6% at 10 years, and 74.9% at 15 years, with an incredibly large variability in the rate of progression to renal death in the different patients.

Using the univariate survivorship analysis described by Kaplan-Maier, we found that the following histological factors influence renal death: more severe intracapillary proliferation, extracapillary proliferation, segmental thickening of the glomerular basement membrane (GBM), glomerular obsolescence, segmental glomerulosclerosis, interstitial fibrosis and arteriolar hyalinosis [2]. That is to say, the more severe the proliferative and sclerotic lesions by light microscopy, the more probable the progression to ESRF. However, the patients with the more severe histological lesions were not necessarily those with a longer duration of the disease.

A significant risk-factor among the immunohistological parameters appeared to be the extension of IgA deposits, outside of the mesangial area, into the wall of peripheral capillary loops [2]. This finding, together with the finding that GBM lesions by light microscopy are also a risk-factor, indicates that the disease is more severe and more susceptible to progress when the deposits and the damage they induce are less restricted to the mesangial area. The cause of this involvement of the peripheral capillary loops is still unknown. Either a more sustained and prolonged overload of immune reactants in the mesangium, with its consequent engulfment and the overflow of complexes to the peripheral capillary walls, or the arrival at the glomerular level of immune complexes of different physicochemical characteristics, which favor entrapment on the subendothelial side of the capillary walls, or a combination of the two, could explain this phenomenon.

The following clinical features appeared to indicate poor prognosis [2]: older age at the onset of the disease; high blood pressure, and considerable proteinuria (these three factors seem to be rather aspecific factors, that apply to all types of glomerular disease).

An additional clinical indicator of poor prognosis that surprised us emerged from our survivorship analysis, and from many similar analyses by other groups: the absence of any history of recurrent macroscopic hematuria (RMH). In other words, the probability of progressing to ESRF is inversely proportional to the number of acute reversible episodes of gross hematuria, usually concomitant with infectious diseases involving the mucosal surfaces: patients without acute clinical exacerbations tend to have a less favorable outcome. There are two possible explanations for this behavior: (1) IgA nephropathy with RMH and IgA nephropathy without RMH are two different diseases, with different severity (some immunogenetic differences tend to confirm this); (2) in the subgroup of patients with RMH, the damaging mechanism, which is identical to that operating in the subgroup without RMH, acts discontinuously (triggered by exogenous antigens coming intermittently from the mucosal surfaces?) while in patients without RMH some less evident but continuously acting immunological mechanism (endogenous antigens?) induces a more severe and progressive damage with time.

Multivariate survivorship analysis of our patients by the regression model of Cox showed that only one clinical variable (proteinuria) and three histological variables (global glomerular sclerosis, interstitial sclerosis and extension of immunodeposits to the peripheral capillary walls) can be considered significant independent predictors of ESRF, global glomerular sclerosis being the most important [2]. Renal survival was 100% when none of the four features was present (32 patients observed for an average postbiopsy period of 4.5 years), and declined to 46.7% when all features were present and glomerular obsolescence was severe (21 patients observed for an average period of 2.4 years).

The fact that glomerular sclerosis and interstitial sclerosis are independent risk factors in IgA nephropathy (even though they appear to be frequently of comparable severity in single patients) seems to us very interesting. We wonder whether interstitial lesions can be induced by or progress independently from the glomerular ones or both. To answer this question, we analyzed interstitial leukocyte infiltration in many patients with IgA nephropathy and found that T lymphocytes were the prevailing infiltrating cells, without any significant modification of the T4+/T8+ ratio, and that the mean members of infiltrating T lymphocytes and also monocytes were greater in a subgroup of patients who had impaired glomerular filtration rate at the time of biopsy, and in patients who, whatever their serum creatinine (SCr) levels at the time of biopsy, showed deterioration of renal function during the post-biopsy follow-up [6].

The characterization of the prevalent infiltrating cells as T lymphocytes, ofter associated with monocytes, obviously suggests that a local cell-mediated immunological mechanism, similar to that which acts in experimental models of tubulointerstitial nephritis and in some cases of human drug-related interstitial nephritis, may be acting in the interstitium in IgA nephropathy. Such a cell-mediated or cytokine-mediated mechanism, even if it is initiated by the same immunological events that act at the glomerulus, or is a consequence of the glomerular damage that such events induce (reaction to unmasked antigens, or cytokines leaking from damaged tissue?), could cause interstitial damage and also contribute to the development of ESRF.

We have said that glomerular sclerosis is the most significant indicator of progression in IgA nephropathy, as it probably is for all glomerular diseases. However, we do not yet know what the mechanisms of its development and progression in Berger's disease are. Three different mechanisms can be proposed: (1) ischemia due to arteriolar lesions; (2) compensatory hyperfiltration of residual nephrons; (3) mesangial overload.

A possible ischemic mechanism has been suggested, because of the morphological pattern (collapse type) and the frequent concomitant finding of arteriolar lesions, even in young patients [7, 8]. However, the correlation between vascular lesions and extent of glomerulosclerosis, which was quite significant ($p < 0.0001$) at the time of biopsy in our total population of 332 patients [2], lost significance in a cohort of patients younger than 45 years whose biopsies were taken early in their disease, when SCr levels were still normal ($p = 0.21$). In this selected group, in which the glomerular obsolescence normally present in older patients should be negligible, glomerulosclerosis was definitely more frequent than vascular damage (60.3 vs 25.4% of patients), suggesting that it can be induced, at least in part, through mechanisms other than ischemia.

We do not believe that compensatory hyperfiltration of residual nephrons is the major responsible factor for the development of glomerular sclerosis in IgA nephropathy, as it is in experimental nephropathies [9], although we cannot exclude that it might favor its accelerated progression in late stages of the disease. Segmental, or even global, glomerular sclerosis can be found in this disease even in early stages, when SCr is still in the normal range and the majority of glomeruli appear morphologically intact by light microscopy. Even as a mechanism of accelerated progression of sclerosis, these hemodynamically mediated changes, if they are operative at all in IgA nephropathy, appear to act at very late stages of functional filtration impairment. The analysis of the rate of progression of renal impairment with time in a subgroup of 77 patients with SCr values between 1.6 and 2.0 mg/dl at the end of a sufficiently long period of observation (2–12 years) indicated a wide range of variability [10]. Twenty-one were rapidly progressing patients who reached ESRF (SCr > 10 mg/dl) within 2 years. In 24 patients the SCr levels were steadly 1.5 to 2 mg/dl in many subsequent determinations and were still less than 2 mg/dl after at least 2 years (5 years for 13 of them, and 8 years for 7). Thus, even after renal damage is already severe enough to cause a pathologic level of SCr, subsequent progression in IgA N is a phenomenon with widely variable velocity. For 20 patients we analyzed a time-series of SCr determinations, subsequent to initial values of SCr from 2.5 to 3.0 mg/100 ml and excluding determinations performed within 2 months after an episode of macroscopic hematuria or acute clinical exacerbation [11]. Even in this group of patients in whom deterioration of renal function was already quite severe at point 0, further progress with time was not a constant phenomenon and some patients had no further deterioration of function for as long as 53 months, in spite of the marked reduction of residual functioning nephrons at point 0.

We favor the hypothesis that in IgA mesangial nephropathy the segmental sclerosis of a progressive number of glomeruli and their subsequent obsolescence are mainly related to the chronic damaging effects of the mesangial overload with IgA immune complexes, and perhaps also other immune complexes, with consequent mesangial matrix overproduction and cell proliferation, 'mesangiolysis', capillary collapse and adhesions to the Bowman's capsule, as has already been demonstrated in some models of experimental nephritis and suggested to be applicable to man.

The four parameters that our multivariate analysis showed to be the most significant indicators of poor prognosis have been used by us to elaborate a score index, to see if we could separate at the time of biopsy those patients who subsequently progress rapidly to ESRF from those with very slow progression [10]. A clear separation was not possible for our population of patients. There was considerable overlap. This means that even those prognostic indicators that appear in the retrospective statistical analysis of a large population of patients to be significant are not always reliable for predicting the outcome for a single patient. In other words, some patients with rather marked proteinuria and/or severe histological lesions at the time of biopsy can have rather favorable courses, and some patients with moderate proteinuria and/or mild histological lesions may have rapidly progressive courses in the following years. This inadequacy of the static picture of the morphological and clinical features at the time of biopsy points once more to the possibility that in IgA nephropathy there may be discontinuous immunological events that temporarily produce additional renal damage during the course of the disease. These could be responsible for the rapidly progressive course that develops in some patients with rather mild lesions at the time of biopsy. On the contrary, if the immunological injurious mechanisms have already stopped acting at the time of biopsy, even patients with advanced proliferative and sclerotic lesions and impairment of renal function may subsequently not progress to more severe renal failure for a long time, even when the number of surviving nephrons is already markedly reduced, as indicated by a large percentage of obsolescent glomeruli by light microscopy and by values of creatinine clearance as low as 30 ml/min. Only when, for a given patient, SCr between 6 and 6.5 mg/dl is selected as the starting point of a sequence of subsequent SCr determinations, is progression a fairly constant phenomenon, but still with different rates for different patients [10].

References

1 D'Amico G, Barbiano di Belgioioso G, Bertoli S, et al: Idiopathic IgA mesangial nephropathy. Clinical and histological study of 374 patients. Medicine 1985;64:49–60.

2 D'Amico G, Minetti L, Ponticelli C, et al: Prognostic indicators in idiopathic IgA mesangial nephropathy. Q J Med 1986;59:363–378.
3 Emancipator SN, Gallo GR, Lamm ME: IgA nephropathy perspectives on pathogenesis and classification. Clin Nephrol 1985;24:161–179.
4 Béné MC, Favre G: IgA nephropathy. Springer Semin Immunopathol 1987;9:387–394.
5 D'Amico G: The commonest glomerulonephritis in the world: IgA nephropathy. Q J Med 1987;64:709–727.
6 Sabadini E, Castiglione A, Colasanti G, et al: Characterization of interstitial infiltrating cells in Berger's disease. Am J Kidney Dis 1988;12:307–315.
7 Clarkson AR, Seymour AE, Thompson AJ, et al: IgA nephropathy: a syndrome of uniform morphology, diverse clinical features and uncertain prognosis. Clin Nephrol 1977;8:549–471.
8 Feiner HD, Cabili S, Baldwin DS, et al: Intrarenal vascular sclerosis in IgA nephropathy. Clin Nephrol 1982;18:183–192.
9 Brenner BM, Meyer TW, Hostetter TH: Dietary protein intake and the progressive nature of kidney disease: The role of hemodynamically mediated glomerular injury in the pathogenesis of progressive glomerular sclerosis in aging, renal ablation, and intrinsic renal disease. N Eng J Med 1982;307:652–659.
10 D'Amico G, Colasanti G, Barbiano di Belgioioso G, et al: Long-term follow-up of IgA mesangial nephropathy: clinico-histological study in 374 patients. Semin Nephrol 1987;7:355–358.
11 Fellin G, Gentile G, Duca G, et al: Renal function in IgA nephropathy with established renal failure. Nephrol Dial Transplant 1988;3:17–23.

Giuseppe D'Amico, MD, Department of Nephrology, S. Carlo Hospital,
Via Pio II, 3, I–20153 Milano (Italy)

Oldrizzi L, Maschio G, Rugiu C, et al. (eds): The Progressive Nature of Renal Disease: Myths and Facts. Contrib Nephrol. Basel, Karger, 1989, vol 75, pp 82–89

The Natural History of Primary Pyelonephritis

Garabed Eknoyan

Renal Section, Department of Medicine, Baylor College of Medicine, Houston, Tex., USA

Shortly after it was recognized that bacterial infection of the urinary tract was a cause of cystitis in 1894, sporadic cases of structural damage of the renal parenchyma and pelvis were reported in patients with severe pyelitis. The appreciation that the 'nephritis' associated with this condition was different from that of glomerular nephritis led the designation of the nephritis attributed to the reaction caused by bacterial invasion of the renal parenchyma as pyelonephritis. The initial reports of such cases were based on the autopsy findings of girls with recurrent urinary tract infections who had died during the course of an acute infection. Later it became clear that there was also a chronic form of pyelonephritis. A causal relationship between pyelonephritis and renal failure was appreciated when Longcope [1] and Weiss and Parker [2] described a group of patients, mostly women aged 15–55 years, with advanced renal failure, many of whom were hypertensive, and had the changes of chronic pyelonephritis at autopsy. The concept then became established that the contracted kidney of chronic pyelonephritis could arise in adults from prior episodes of infection of the kidney. The onset of the disease was assumed to be due to acute pyelonephritis, which then progressed insidiously to renal failure, over a period of 10–15 years, despite a generally sterile urine after the initial episode of infection. It was evident from the outset that some form of obstruction to both ureters predisposed the kidneys to infection and that in rare instances there was congenital stricture or unexplained dilatation of the ureters [1]. However, in most of the cases there was little or no evident obstruction, and this group was identified as having chronic nonobstructive pyelonephritis.

Prompted by the identification of this new cause of renal failure, retrospective reviews of major autopsy series which appeared in the 1950s and early 1960s began to report an increasing incidence of pyelonephritis (table 1). Threatened by the failure to have diagnosed antemortem what

Table 1. Autopsy incidence of pyelonephritis reported in the literature

	Year	Incidence, %	Number of cases
Lancet ii:903	1928	6	1,800
NEJM 217:725	1937	2	2,043
Renal Disease	1948	5.6	3,607
Med Clin North Am 39:297	1955	9.0	4,425
NEJM 256:915	1957	8.1	5,000
Geriatrics 14:25	1959	20	900
Medicine 39:3	1960	15	4,193
Arch Intern Med 105:23	1960	9.6	11,157
Am J Med 30:589	1961	2.8	3,393
Bull NY Acad Med 37:367	1961	12	2,991
Am J Dis Child 104:215	1962	1.6	1,999
Ann Intern Med 66:697	1967	1.4	4,686
		$\bar{x}$ 7.8	46,194

was taunted as a common cause of renal failure at autopsy, there emerged an increasing propensity to attribute to chronic pyelonephritis any apparently causeless instance of chronic renal failure and hypertension encountered clinically, especially in the presence of a disparity in the size of the two kidneys on urography. The initial epidemiologic studies following the introduction of quantitative bacteriologic urine cultures fueled this proclivity to diagnose chronic pyelonephritis, particularly when it became apparent that a significant portion of the population had organisms in the urine and that some of these bacteriuric individuals were asymptomatic [3, 4]. However, the majority of these were female, a finding inconsistent with the autopsy reports in which the lesions of pyelonephritis were noted to be as common in males as in females. The establishment of strict morphologic criteria of postmortem diagnosis, coupled by the appreciation of other causes of tubulointerstitial disease, soon led to the reversal of the reported incidence of pyelonephritis diagnosed at postmortem examination of the kidney (table 1). In fact, it was probably the appreciation of the lesions of analgesic abuse that had the greatest impact in questioning the wisdom of attributing all tubulointerstitial lesions to pyelonephritis [5]. Furthermore, it became evident from the study of patients coming to dialysis and transplantation that pyelonephritis was not the commonest cause of end-stage kidney disease [6]. The impact has been a gradual reduction in the tendency to diagnose pyelonephritis (fig. 1).

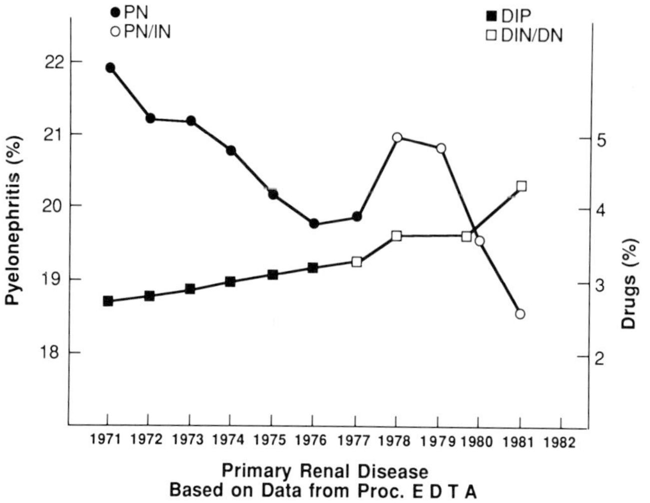

Fig. 1. Percent of cases with end-stage renal disease in which pyelonephritis was considered the primary renal disease. Based on data reported in volumes 8 through 18 of the Proceedings of the European Dialysis and Transplant Association. PN = Pyelonephritis; PN/IN = pyelonephritis/interstitial nephritis; DIP = drug-induced pyelonephritis; DIN/DN = drug-induced nephropathy/drug nephropathy.

Cross-sectional and prospective studies have now revealed that silent renal destructive cases of pyelonephritis are clinically much less common than had been postulated and that in cases with recurrent symptomatic urinary tract infection impairment of renal function may be difficult to spot [3, 4]. The demonstration of vesicoureteral reflux (VUR) in children with symptomatic bacteriuria and the observation that the highest incidence of focal renal scarring occurred in those with severe VUR has resulted in a remarkable shift in the emphasis of the role of primary pyelonephritis as a cause of progressive renal failure [3, 4, 7, 8]. It has become evident from several studies that chronic focal pyelonephritis is predominantly an entity limited to children, occurs mostly during the first 2 years of age and seldom arises later in life, particularly passed the age of ten [3]. There is now incontrovertible evidence from many sources that the presence of VUR renders a child with recurrent infections liable to progressive renal damage. Depending on the severity of the VUR and the frequency of the infectious episodes this will result in renal failure during the early years of life, but only in a few of these individuals. The majority of cases remain symptomless and in good health during subsequent childhood and early adult life, though subject to reinfection, notably with pregnancy. Furthermore, despite the fact that urographic abnormalities may become evident in some, the development of hypertension and renal failure is extremely uncommon in them [3, 4, 7, 8]. Prospective studies have shown that the infected kidney is slow to mature but is well compensated for by hypertrophy of the contralateral kidney, and that a conspicuous growth spurt of the scarred kidney occurs at puberty, sometimes a decade after the original injury, particularly if the urine is kept sterile [9, 10]. From the available literature the following still hazy picture of the course of events seems to emerge. Continued urinary tract infection in childhood is likely to produce progressive radiographic evidence of focal renal parenchymal injury, particularly in the presence of VUR. Most of these cases have normal renal function in early adult life, although pyelonephritis of pregnancy and toxemia appear to be more common in them. A smaller group progresses to renal failure, usually with hypertension in early middle life, i.e. well after 15–20 years following the initial episodes of acute pyelonephritis. Early diagnosis of infectious episodes and their appropriate treatment will arrest the development and progression of renal changes.

Thus, the general proposition that pyelonephritis can lead to renal injury and failure is both reasonable and supported by the available evidence. However, to the extent that this occurs in the presence of VUR renders the course and, in fact, the validity of primary pyelonephritis, questionable. The sense of guilt created by this evidence has led to a counterreaction in the use of the term 'pyelonephritis' in the recent nephrology literature. In the latest edition of 'Diseases of the Kidney', the term 'chronic pyelonephritis' does not appear in the title of the chapter discussing it which is labelled 'Infections of the Upper Urinary Tract' [11]; while perusal of the index of 'The Kidney' refers the searcher for chronic pyelonephritis to VUR [12].

This may well be a premature overreaction. Firstly, whereas it is true that the application of stricter criteria to the diagnosis of pyelonephritis has resulted in a significant reduction in the incidence of pyelonephritis, pyelonephritis remains a common cause of renal failure. In fact in the very study that first applied these criteria and noted that less than 3% of the 3,000 autopsied cases had pyelonephritis, with less than 20% of them dying of uremia, of the 100 deaths in uremia 57% had pyelonephritis [13].

Secondly, autopsy studies have shown that in addition to the classic irregularly contracted kidney of childhood, a second type of diffuse evenly contracted kidneys, one being smaller than the other, occurs in adults in whom destruction of the parenchyma appears to occur without localized scarring. The course of such a sequence of events is substantiated from the report of cases encountered clinically, where the evolution of the changes was evaluated radiographically and occurred in the absence of documented obstruction or reflux [14, 15]. The argument that in such cases VUR has subsided, was mild or undemonstrable becomes circuitous and self-serving [8].

Thirdly, the close correlation between renal scarring and VUR is based mainly on studies emanating from referral centers [7, 10]. It does not seem to be supported by prospective studies. In one such study, among 23 kidneys in which renal scars developed during follow-up, severe (grade III and IV) reflux was present at the time of infection in only one third of the cases. In the others there was either grade II reflux (26%) or no reflux (39%) [10]. To the extent that experimental urinary tract infection has been shown to cause ureteritis with ureteral paralysis [16], which could be associated with functional reflux, the role of primary infection may well have been discounted prematurely in some cases.

Fourthly, the fact that VUR is much more common that childhood urinary tract infection has been documented in relatives of symptomatic children, and when uncomplicated by infection appears to subside by the first decade of life without any evidence of detrimental effects on renal function. It would seem evident then that the presence of infection appears to be important for VUR to exert a detrimental effect on the kidney. Coupled by the albeit rare cases of primary infection, without evidence of VUR, associated with renal damage, it is fair to conclude that it is infection rather than VUR that is detrimental to kidney function and initiates the sequence of events that leads to progressive renal failure [10, 17]. A similar argument can be made for some of the other causes of renal failure in which the renal lesions are those of chronic tubulointerstitial nephropathy. The study that has been most widely quoted in support of the argument that infection uncomplicated by other factors is relatively rare as a cause of end-stage renal disease is that of Murray and Goldberg [18]. In this report of 101 patients with chronic renal insufficient attributed to chronic interstitial nephritis, 27% had bacterial infections but all of them had an associated primary cause of their renal disease. The diagnosis of interstitial nephritis in this study was a clinical one and not substantiated by actual morphology. In a series of 48 biopsy documented cases of tubulointerstitial nephropathy we studied, urine cultures were positive in 23% of them. Other reports substantiate that infection occurs rather frequently (20–25%) in patients with renal failure [19]. In a subset of those associated with obstruction (stones, VUR) and vascular disease (diabetes, sickle cell disease), infection appears to contribute to the progression of renal failure. Whether the presence of infection contributes to the progression of other kidney diseases cannot be ascertained, but is a distinct possibility. In fact, in diseases in which infection seems to play a contributory role to the progression of renal failure, the lesions appear to be more prominent in the

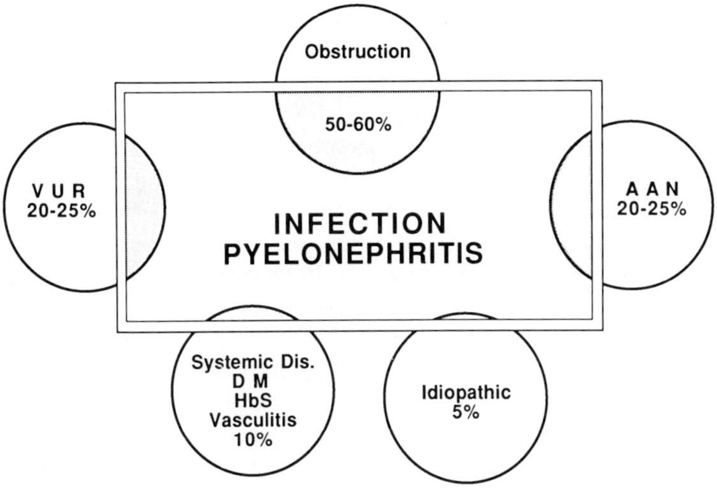

Fig. 2. Spectrum of diseases in which renal parenchymal infection (pyelonephritis) contributes to the deterioration of kidney function. VUR = Vesicoureteral reflux; AAN = analgesic abuse nephropathy; DM = diabetes mellitus; HbS = sickle cell hemoglobinopathy.

medulla and result in papillary necrosis. In a report of 27 cases, infection was present in 18 or two thirds of them [20]. In 14 of the 18 cases, there was another identifiable cause of papillary necrosis, and the infection was considered a secondary factor. It was proposed, therefore, that the pathogenesis of renal papillary necrosis represents an overlap phenomenon of more than one factor with infection playing an important contributory role. A similar scheme can be presented for the role of pyelonephritis in progressive renal failure (fig. 2). In this scheme primary pyelonephritis contributes only to a small number of cases. More importantly, VUR, although an important contributory cause, is not the sole entity associated with the progressive renal lesions of chronic pyelonephritis. Obstruction, analgesic abuse nephropathy, and systemic diseases that are associated with vasculopathy appear to be equally important and common. To equate the renal lesions of chronic pyelonephritis with VUR alone [12] is much too restrictive and inconsistent with the available evidence.

The rate of progression to renal failure in the presence of pyelonephritis is hard to determine. From a study of the incidence and pattern of chronic renal failure in adults observed during a period of 5 years in Gothenburg, Sweden [21], pyelonephritis was present in 52 of the 145 patients who progressed to end-stage renal disease, from the time of diagnosis of renal insufficiency (creatinine >5 mg/100 ml). It was the most common cause, followed in sequential order by glomerulonephritis, diabetes mellitus, polycystic kidney disease, nephrosclerosis and amyloidosis. About one third (36%) of the patients diagnosed as pyelonephritis had non-obstructive pyelonephritis and the remainder (63%) had analgesic abuse nephropathy. The mean duration to end-stage renal disease in these 52 patients was 13.6 months (range 0.7–52.4 months), which ranked fifth in the order of rapidity of progression, being preceded by amyloidosis ($\bar{x}$ 5.3 months), nephrosclerosis ($\bar{x}$ 5.7 months), diabetes mellitus ($\bar{x}$ 6 months), and glomerulonephritis ($\bar{x}$ 10.1 months). Polycystic kidney disease was the slowest to progress to end-stage renal disease ($\bar{x}$ 18.1 months).

Thus, it would seem that once renal insufficiency develops, the disease seems to be progressive [21–23]. Assuming the generally accepted rate of deterioration of the glomerular filtration rate in diabetes of 1–1.2 ml/months, and given the length of time to develop end-stage renal disease of these two groups in the study from Gothenburg [21], the rate of deterioration of glomerular filtration rate in pyelonephritis can be projected to be about 0.5 ml/min. Obviously, this is a speculative figure, based on one study of cases that included analgesic abuse nephropathy. Naturally, the figure would vary from case to case, particularly in the presence of other complications.

References

1 Longcope WT: Chronic bilateral pyelonephritis: Its origin and its association with hypertension. Ann Intern Med 1937;11:149–163.

2 Weiss S, Parker F: Pyelonephritis: Its relation to vascular lesions and to arterial hypertension. Medicine 1939;18:221–315.

3 MacGregor M: Pyelonephritis lenta. Consideration of childhood urinary infection as the forerunner of renal insufficiency in later life. Arch Dis Child 1970;45:159–172.

4 Kunin CM: Does kidney infection cause renal failure? Annu Rev Med 1985;36:165–176.

5 Eknoyan G: Chronic tubulointerstitial nephropathies; in Schrier RW, Gottschalk CW (eds): Diseases of the Kidney, ed 4. Boston, Little, Brown, 1988.

6 Gault MH, Dossetor JB: Chronic pyelonephritis: Relative incidence in transplant recipients. N Engl J Med 1966;275:813–816.

7 Hodson CJ, Edwards D: Chronic pyelonephritis and vesicoureteric reflux. Clin Radiol 1960;11:219–228.

8 Thomsen HS, Dorph S: Caliceal clubbing and adjacent parenchymal scarring (always reflux nephropathy?) as a cause of end-stage renal failure. Acta Radiol [Diag] 1986;27:705–710.

9 Claesson I, Jacobsson B, Jodal U, et al: Compensatory kidney growth in children with urinary tract infection and unilateral renal scarring: An epidemiologic study. Kidney Int 1981;20:759–764.

10 Winberg J, Bollgren I, Kallenius G, et al: Clinical pyelonephritis and focal renal scarring. A selected review of pathogenesis, prevention and prognosis. Pediatr Clin North Am 1982;29:801–814.

11 Ronald AR, Simonsen JN: Infections of the upper urinary tract; in Schrier RW, Gottschalk CW (eds): Diseases of the Kidney, ed 4. Boston, Little, Brown, 1988.
12 de Wardner HE: The Kidney, ed 5. Edinburgh, Churchill-Livingstone, 1985.
13 Kimmelstiel P: Significance of chronic pyelonephritis; in Quinn EL, Kass EH (eds): Biology of Pyelonephritis. Boston, Little, Brown, 1960, pp 215–224.
14 Bailey RR, Little PJ, Rolleston GL: Renal damage after acute pyelonephritis. Br Med J 1969;i:550–551.
15 Davies AG, McLachlan MSF, Asscher AW: Progressive kidney damage after non-obstructive urinary tract infection. Br Med J 1972;i:406–407.
16 Roberts JA: Experimental pyelonephritis in the monkey. III. Pathophysiology of ureteral malfunction induced by bacteria. Invest Urol 1975;13:117–122.
17 Hostetter TH, Nath KA, Hostetter MK: Infection-related chronic interstitial nephropathy. Semin Nephrol 1988–8:11–16.
18 Murray T, Goldberg M: Chronic interstitial nephritis: Etiologic factors. Ann Intern Med 1975;82:453–459.
19 Leonard CD, Cutter RE, Johnson JT, et al: Bacteriuria in noninfectious renal disease. Am J Med Sci 1969;258:230–236.
20 Eknoyan G, Qunibi WY, Grissom RT, et al: Renal papillary necrosis: An update. Medicine 1982;61:55–73.
21 Ahlmen J: Incidence of chronic renal insufficiency. A study of the incidence and pattern of renal insufficiency in adults during 1966–1971 in Gothenburg. Acta Med Scand 1975(Suppl 582):1–50.
22 Angell ME, Relman AS, Robbins SL: 'Active' chronic pyelonephritis without evidence of bacterial infection. N Engl J Med 1968;278:1303–1308.
23 Huland H, Busch R: Chronic pyelonephritis as a cause of end-stage renal disease. J Urol 1982;127:642–643.

Garabed Eknoyan, MD, Department of Medicine, Baylor College of Medicine,
One Baylor Plaza, Houston, TX 77030 (USA)

Oldrizzi L, Maschio G, Rugiu C, et al. (eds): The Progressive Nature of Renal Disease: Myths and Facts. Contrib Nephrol. Basel, Karger, 1989, vol 75, pp 90–99

The Natural History of Reflux Nephropathy

Pietro Zucchelli, Rossella Gaggi, Alessandro Zuccalà

Divisione di Nefrologia e Dialisi Malpighi, Ospedale S. Orsola Malpighi, USL 28, Bologna, Italia

Primary vesico-ureteric reflux (VUR) is a congenital abnormality mainly caused by incompetence of the uretero-vesical junction in the absence of bladder outlet obstruction, neurovesical dysfunction, etc. [1]. In children, the frequency, clinical presentation and diagnosis of VUR are well-known and documented [2]. In adults, the clinical importance of VUR is particularly related to the consequences of the reflux extention into the pyelotubular system, leading to the development of the VUR complication called reflux nephropathy (RN). RN is mainly a radiological term which describes a particular kind of chronic pyelonephritis with scarring, contraction and distortion of renal architecture: it is usually diagnosed by intravenous urography, as reported in table 1 [3]. RN may be an important cause of chronic renal failure and in some centers it is almost certainly under-diagnosed [4–6].

The aim of this study is to describe and analyze our experience of RN in adults and collect data on the clinical manifestations, prognosis and outcome of this disease.

Patients and Clinical Data

Between 1976 and 1987, 95 patients (32 males and 63 females) were diagnosed in our department as having primary RN. The mean age at the first examination was 32.2 years (range 15–63 years) and the mean interval between the first signs or symptoms and the diagnosis was 9.1 years, ranging between 6 months and 40 years. The diagnosis was established before the age of 12 in only 10 patients (10%). All the patients satisfied the radiographic selection criteria reported in table 1 [7]. The 95 patients represented 1.3% of all new patients admitted to our department during the same period (as an indirect comparison of the frequency, membranous nephropathy corresponded to an incidence of 2.9% of the new patients). RN was present in all but one patient, unilaterally in 32 patients (33.7%) and bilaterally in 62 patients (66.3%). The urographic classification of RN, according to Smellie et al. [8], is reported in figure 1. We found no correlation between the grade of reflux and the

Table 1. Diagnosis criteria

High-dose intravenous urography with tomography Calyceal clubbing and adjacent cortical scarring Arrest of renal growth especially at polar site Ureteral dilatation
Micturating cystourethrography VUR passive at different degrees of bladder distension or active during micturation
Exclusion of secondary VUR

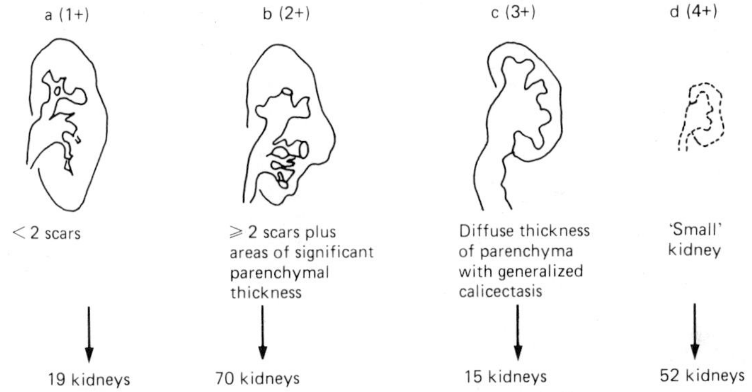

Fig. 1. Urographic classification of reflux nephropathy. Grade frequency in our 95 patients. From ref. [8].

extent of progressive scarring in adults. RN may include different types of clinical presentation: urinary tract infection (UTI), hypertension, loin pain, urinary calculi, proteinuria and renal failure. The main reasons for the first nephrological examination are reported in table 2. Hence, quite unlike what occurs during childhood, urinary tract symptoms are not commonly responsible for the diagnosis in adulthood. However, a careful analysis of the clinical history reveals the presence of UTI or episodic loin pain and/or fever in approximately half of the patients, as shown in table 3. Table 3 also shows that the first symptoms or signs of RN in women often appeared during pregnancy, sometimes mimicking preeclampsia in the first or second trimester. Moreover, women with RN may develop a variety of complications during pregnancy, as shown in table 4. Judging from those clinical data there is little doubt of that in many adult patients. RN is manifested with recurrent UTI or with other related symptoms during childhood or during pregnancy. On the other hand, it appears that many newly diagnosed adult patients with RN never had UTI in infancy or early childhood. The absence of any urinary tract symptoms could mislead the clinician into delaying diagnosis [6].

Table 2. Main reason for the first nephrological investigation

	Male	Female	All patients	%
Renal failure	12	12	24	25.3
Asymptomatic proteinuria	8	13	21	22.1
Urinary tract symptoms	3	18	21	22.1
Hematuria	5	8	13	13.6
Hypertension	3	8	11	11.4
Recurrent fever	–	3	3	3.3
Nephrolithiasis	1	1	2	2.2

Table 3. Clinical history – frequency of complaints

	Male	Female	All patients	
			number	%
Lower urinary tract symptoms[1]	4	22	26	27.3
Loin pain[1]	5	22	27	28.4
Recurrent fever[1]	7	18	25	26.3
Painful hematuria (macroscopic)	10 (5)	14 (3)	24 (8)	25.2
Proteinuria	5	12	17	17.9
Hypertension	3	8	11	11.5
Asymptomatic bacteriuria	–	7	7	7.3
Nephrolitiasis	1	1	2	2.2
Enuresis or daytime incontinence	–	2	2	2.2
Renal failure	3	2	5	5.2

[1] Symptoms appeared during pregnancy in approximately 25% of all the female patients.

Table 4. Vesico-ureteric reflux and complications during pregnancy[1]

	Number of patients	% of pregnancies
Urinary tract symptoms	13	18.1
Hypertension	8	11.1
Proteinuria	14	19.4
Preeclampsia (EPH gestosis)	9	12.4
Miscarriage	3	4.1
Deterioration in renal function	3	4.1
In utero fetal death	1	1.3
Still-born death	1	1.3

[1] Out of 40 women with a total of 72 pregnancies, 37 (51%) were complication-free, whereas 35 (49%) suffered from complications.

Table 5. Symptom frequency at diagnosis

	Patients with UT symptoms (%)	Patients without UT symptoms (%)	p
Patients	60 (63)	35 (37)	
Male/female	14/46	18/17	<0.01
Proteinuria > 200 mg/24 h	25 (41.6)	27 (77.1)	<0.005
SCr > 1.5 mg/dl	20 (33.3)	22 (62.6)	<0.005
Males with renal failure	6	17	
Hypertension	14 (23.3)	18 (51.4)	<0.05

Table 6. Incidence of various signs according to sex

	Males (%)	Females (%)	p
Patients	32	63	
Proteinuria	27 (84.3)	25 (39.7)	<0.001
Renal failure	23 (71.9)	19 (30.1)	<0.001
Hypertension	12 (37.5)	20 (31.7)	n.s.

$p = \chi^2$ test.

Sex as a Prognostic Index

We have subdivided our patients into two groups, according to the presence or absence of a clinical history which points to VUR (table 5). The frequency of the various signs corresponds to the whole population at the last control. RN is more often associated with UT symptoms in female patients, whereas male patients more frequently have an asymptomatic follow-up with the subsequent appearance of proteinuria, hematuria or renal failure.

Sex seems to be an important factor in the formation of severe scars and in progressive disease, as pointed out by Kincaid-Smith [9]. In our study, male patients have a significantly higher frequency of proteinuria and renal failure but not hypertension (blood pressure more than 150/90 mm/Hg) than female ones (table 6).

Many authors have stressed the importance of infection in inducing scar formations and growth arrest during infancy. In adults, on the other hand, the association of newly diagnosed severe RN and sterile urine with no history of UTI seems to go against the theory that urinary infection is an essential prerequisite for scarring formation, according to the Big-Bang hypothesis [10].

Table 7. Eighty patients were followed up for a mean period of 5.7 years (range 2–14 years)

	Number of patients	Renal failure, %
Patients with proteinuria < 200 mg/day	30	10
Patients with proteinuria > 200 mg–1 gr/day	27	59
Patients with proteinuria < 1 –3 g/day	16	87
Patients with proteinuria > 3 g/day	7	100

Table 8. Vesico-ureteric reflux and hypertension

	Patients with hypertension (%)	Patients without hypertension (%)
Hypertension evident at first examination (95 patients)	21 (22.1)	
Malignant hypertension	1 (1.1)	
Last control (80 patients)		
Number	28 (35)	52 (65)
With renal failure	16 (57)	24 (46)
Males with renal failure	8	13

Natural History of Reflux Nephropathy

Eighty of our 95 patients were followed up for at least 2 years and for a mean period of 5.6 years (ranging from 2 to 14 years). Both the presence and the amount of proteinuria certainly represent the major prognostic indices, since renal failure was observed in only 10% of the patients without significant proteinuria and in all the patients with nephrotic-range proteinuria (table 7). As concerns hypertension, the present data confirm our previous results [7], i.e. that it occurred more frequently in RN patients than in the unselected population. Hypertension is usually benign and rarely follows a malignant course (table 8). In our series, hypertension was definitely more frequent in patients with renal failure than in those without, but the difference was not very high and progression to chronic renal failure may even be observed in many patients with normal blood pressure.

Table 9. Main characteristics of groups I-III

	Group I	Group II	Group III
Patients	40	24	16
Male/female	8/32	12/12	9/7
Mean SCr at first examination, mg/dl	1.39 (0.8–1.7)	2.58 (1.0–6.3)	2.24 (0.9–6.8)
Bilateral reflux nephropathy, %	40	100	100
UTI, %	70	58.3	50
Hypertension, %	30	37.5	43
Mean follow-up, months	67 ± 34	75 ± 35	51 ± 27

The rate of renal function decline over time (months) in the 80 patients was analyzed by least squares linear regression, according to the following formula [11]:

$$[\Sigma_i x, y, -((\Sigma_i x, \Sigma_i y,)/n))/(\Sigma_i x^2, -(\Sigma_i x,)^2/n)],$$

where x = months of follow-up; y = 1/serum creatinine (1/SCr); n = number of observations.

Among the 80 patients, the ones whose graph of reciprocal SCr against time was clearly nonlinear by inspection were excluded. The patients were then subdivided into 3 groups: group I – no progression; group II – slow deterioration of renal function and a regression coefficient less than – 0.004; group III – a more rapid deterioration of renal function and a regression coefficient between −0.004 and −0.02. The main characteristics of the 3 groups are reported in table 9. Patients who did not have a deterioration in renal function during the follow-up were more often female with a higher incidence of UTI; they more frequently had unilateral RN with SCr at first examination less than 1.7 mg/dl. Hypertension in stable patients was a less frequent occurrence than in those who deteriorated, although there was no clear-cut statistical difference. Moreover, significant proteinuria was uncommon in the former with a significantly lower grade of renal scarring compared to those who progressed. Renal insufficiency only occurred in patients with bilateral scars. More interestingly, the sex, the grades of scarring (fig. 2), the initial SCr, the frequency of hypertension and UTI did not appear to influence the renal function

2
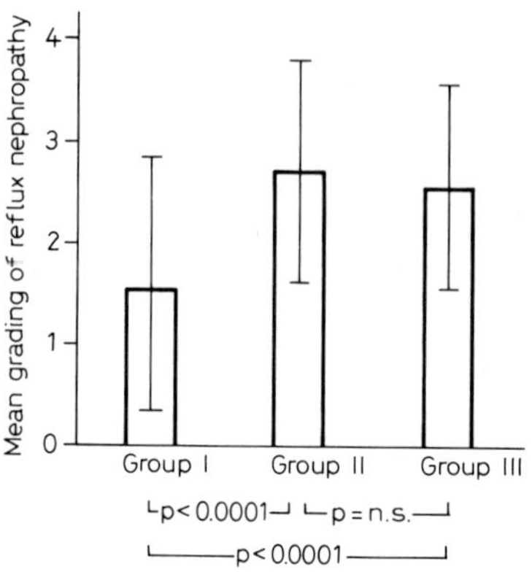

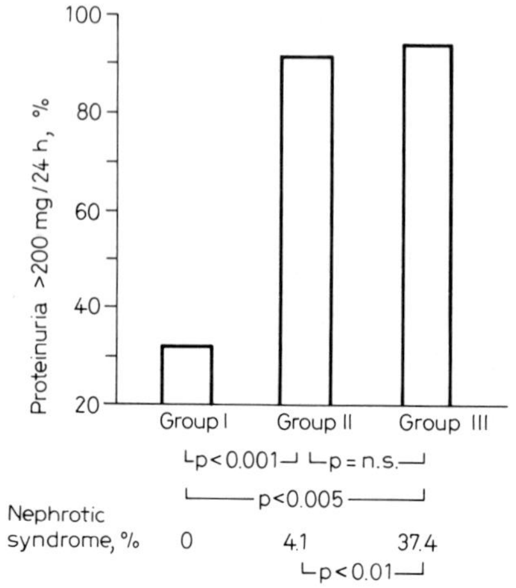

3

Fig. 2. Mean values (and SD) of the reflux nephropathy grades in stable patients (group I), in patients with slow deterioration of renal function (group II) and with more rapid deterioration (group III).

Fig. 3. Mean values of proteinuria frequency in stable patients (group I), in patients with slow deterioration of renal function (group II) and with more rapid deterioration (group III).

deterioration rate. Only the amount of proteinuria significantly distinguished group II from group III patients. Indeed, nephrotic range proteinuria was significantly more frequent in group III than in group II (fig. 3).

All our patients were advised to assume a low-protein diet (0.6–0.7 g/kg body weight). Owing to the retrospective nature of this work, we have no objective data on the patient compliance to the diet. However, in a small but carefully followed up group of 18 RN patients with a SCr over 2.2 mg/dl, the compliance to a low-protein diet of 46 ± 12 g/day was confirmed for at least one year by 24-hour urinary urea excretion. All patients received antihypertensive treatment with conventional drugs. The different progression rate in the latter group of patients showed no correlation to protein intake. The mean values of proteinuria (1.12 ± 0.6 g/24 h in patients with slow progression versus 1.93 ± 0.7 g/24 h in patients with a higher progression rate) and blood pressure (fig. 4) were the only differences between the two groups.

Twenty-five patients were operated on for VUR (table 10). Unilateral nephrectomy was suggested for atrophic pyelonephritic kidney associated to gross VUR and persistent UTI. Surgical correction of the reflux, successfully performed in 17 patients, seemed to reduce the incidence of UTI episodes, although the fate of renal function was unaffected.

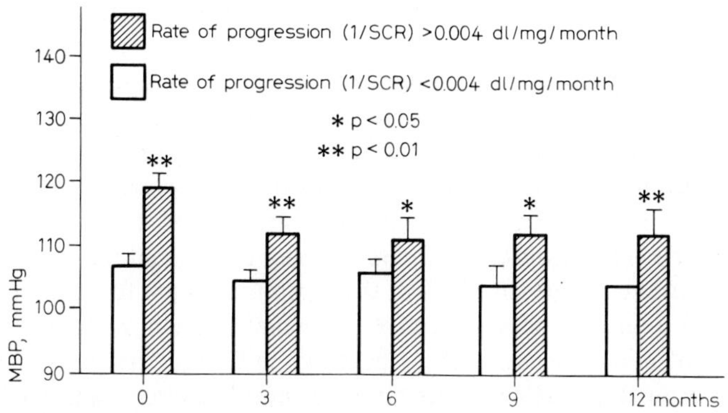

Fig. 4. Mean values of mean blood pressure (MBP) in patients with different rate of renal insufficiency progression.

Table 10. Surgery in vesico-ureteric reflux

Patients	25	
Mean age (range), years	23 (16–38)	
Unilateral nephrectomies	8	
Ureteric reimplantations	17	
	Pre-surgery	Post-surgery
UTI	13	8
Hypertension	3	7
Proteinuria > 200 mg/day	9	10
Renal failure	7	8

Finally, 15 of our 95 patients reached end-stage renal failure, corresponding to 2.9% of our dialysis population. The mean age at the start of the dialysis program was 29.2 years (range 18–44) in males and 37.4 years (range 17–58) in females.

Comments and Conclusions

VUR, and especially its main complication, i.e. reflux nephropathy, represents a fairly frequent disease in adults. RN is often associated to recurrent UTI during childhood or pregnancy in female patients, even though it appears that renal scarring may also be caused by the intrarenal reflux of sterile urine. Male patients more often have an asymptomatic follow-up with late appearance of proteinuria and/or renal failure. Both the presence and the amount of proteinuria represent the major prognostic indices. It is now well-known that focal and segmental glomerulosclerosis (FSG) is very common in RN [9, 12, 13]. FSG has also been documented in 5 of our proteinuric patients in whom we performed transcutaneous renal biopsy. Our study suggests that there is a degree of renal failure which inevitably leads to the progressive loss of the remaining renal function, even if the underlying disease process is removed. In fact, the elimination of the primary causes of renal disease, such as bacteria and reflux, are not able to modify progression when SCr is more than 1.7 mg/dl and/or bilateral RN (with severe renal scarring) is present. The destruction of a specifically defined nephron population leaves the remaining nephrons vulnerable to the appearance of FSG. In our study, there is no data supporting any of the various mechanisms which might be involved in the genesis of the glomerular lesions [9, 14, 15]. However, regardless of the pathogenesis of FSG, its strong association with RN brings to mind the issue of sex. Indeed, male patients with RN have a more serious progression compared to female ones. Renal ablation in rats [15] and humans [16] results in the development of proteinuria and FSG much sooner in males than in similar females.

Hypertension is certainly more frequent in RN patients with renal failure than in those without, but the presence of high blood pressure does not seem to have a clear-cut detrimental effect on this type of diseased kidney. Blood pressure under conventional therapy was significantly lower only in a selected group of carefully followed up patients with reduced rates of progression than in those with a higher progression rate. There may be two possible explanations for the difference in the progression rates between these two groups of patients: one possibility is that the reduction in blood pressure may have a beneficial effect on intraglomerular hemodynamics; the other is that a more severe form of RN also accounts for some types of 'refractory' hypertension.

References

1 Lyon RP, Marshall S, Tanagho EA: The ureteral orifice: its configuration and competency. J Urol 1969;102:504–509.

2 Smellie JM, Normand ICS: Reflux nephropathy in childhood; in Hodson CJ, Kincaid Smith P (ed): Reflux Nephropathy, New York, Masson, 1979, pp 14–18.

3 Hodson CJ, Edwards D: Chronic pyelonephritis and vesico-ureteral reflux. Clin Radiol 1960;11:219–331.

4 Bailey RR: End stage reflux nephropathy. Nephron 1981;27:302–306.

5 Salvatierra OJR, Tanagho EA: Reflux as a cause of end stage kidney disease: reported of 32 cases. J Urol 1977;117:441–443.
6 Bailey RR: Clinical presentation and diagnosis of vesico-ureteric reflux nephropathy; in Davison AM, Briggs JD, Green R, Kanis JA, Mallick NP, Rees AJ, Thomson D (eds): Nephrology. London, Baillière, Tindall, 1988, vol II, pp 835–843.
7 Zucchelli P, Gaggi R: Vesico ureteral reflux and reflux nephropathy in adults. Contrib Nephrol 1988;61:210–219.
8 Smellie JM, Edwards D, Hunter N, et al: Vesico-ureteric reflux and renal scarring. Kidney Int 1975;8:65–72.
9 Kincaid-Smith PS: Natural history and treatment of reflux nephropathy; in Robinson RR, Dennis VW, Ferris TF, Glassock RJ, Kokko JP, Tisher CC (eds): Nephrology. New York, Springer, 1988, vol II, pp 958–979.
10 Ransley PG, Risdon RA: Reflux nephropathy: Effects of antimicrobial therapy on the evolution of the early pyelonephritic scar. Kidney Int 1981;20:733–742.
11 Mitch WE, Walser M: A simple method of estimating progression of chronic renal failure. Lancet 1976;ii:1326–1328.
12 Bhatema DB, Weiss JH, Holland NH, et al: Focal and segmental glomerular sclerosis in reflux nephropathy. Am J Med 1980;68:886–892.
13 Torres EV, Velosa JA, Holley EKP, et al: The progression of vesico-ureteral reflux nephropathy. Ann Intern Med 1980;92:776–784.
14 Brenner BM: Hemodynamically mediated glomerular injury and the progressive nature of kidney disease. Kidney Int 1983;23:647–655.
15 Elema JD, Arends A: Focal and segmental glomerular hyalinosis and sclerosis in the rat. Lab Invest 1976;33:554–561.
16 Zucchelli P, Cagnoli L, Casanova S, et al: Focal glomerulosclerosis in patients with unilateral nephrectomy. Kidney Int 1983;24:649–655.

Prof. Pietro Zucchelli, Divisione de Nefrologia e Dialisi Malpighi,
Policlinico S. Orsola-Malpighi, Via P. Palagi 9, I–40138 Bologna (Italy)

Oldrizzi L, Maschio G, Rugiu C, et al. (eds): The Progressive Nature of Renal Disease: Myths and Facts. Contrib Nephrol. Basel, Karger, 1989, vol 75, pp 100–107

The Natural History of Inherited Renal Diseases

Jean-Michel Pochet[a], *Ginette Albouze*[b], *Guillaume Bobrie*[a], *Paul Landais*[c], *Christiane Ferran*[a], *Jean-Pierre Grünfeld*[a]

[a] Département de Néphrologie, Hôpital Necker; [b] Centre d'Hémodialyse, Chateauroux; [c] Laboratoire de Biostatistique et d'Informatique Médicale, Hôpital Necker, Paris, France

Among inherited kidney diseases observed in adults, autosomal dominant polycystic kidney disease (ADPKD) and Alport's syndrome (and related nephropathies) are the most frequent. We will focus on the rate of progression of renal failure in these two diseases. The natural history of these inherited disorders provides the opportunity of evaluating the respective part and interplay of genetic and environmental factors in the progression of the renal involvement. Genetic heterogeneity should also be taken into account.

Progression of Renal Failure in Autosomal Dominant Polycystic Kidney Disease

ADPKD is well known by nephrologists since it represents approximately 10% of all causes of end-stage renal failure (ESRF) in Western countries. The mean age at first dialysis is approximately 50 years [1]. In our center, between 1972 and 1987, 138 ADPKD patients went to regular dialysis, which was initiated between 40 and 59 years in 76%, before 40 years in 4% and after 59 years in 20% of them.

It should be kept in mind, however, that a substantial number of ADPKD patients do not progress or progress more slowly to renal failure. In the study by Iglesias et al. [2], the diagnosis of ADPKD was made at autopsy in 16 cases, including 8 patients who died at 80 years of age or more. In a population-based assessment, Churchill et al. [3] have stated that the probability for ADPKD subjects of being alive without ESRF was 77% by age 50 and 52% by age 73. Conversely, ADPKD may be detected in infancy and early progression to renal failure has been observed [4].

The relationship between the rate of growth of renal cysts and the renal prognosis has not been well delineated. It has been suggested that cysts develop in relatively few nephrons and collecting ducts and that impairment of renal function is proportional to the growth of the established cysts, which compress adjacent parenchyma [5]. This view has recently been challenged [1]. It is supported, however, by the data of Gabow et al. [6] who showed that the number of renal cysts did not relate to the serum creatinine concentration but that the size of the cysts did. This view might also justify surgical or pharmacological attempts to reduce early cyst size. Whether slowly progressive ADPKD is characterized by slow growth of cysts or by a lower percentage of affected nephrons is presently unknown. Histological examinations of kidneys from ADPKD patients who do not progress to renal failure would be of great interest in this regard.

What are the other factors potentially involved in determining the rate of progression?

Genetic Factors. The ADPKD locus has been located on the short arm of chromosome 16 by using several DNA probes [7]. Recently, no linkage with these probes was found in two ADPKD families of Italian origin [8]. Apparently, the progression is not different from that observed in classical ADPKD.

The rate of progression is often heterogeneous within a given family. In some unusual kindreds with slowly progressive ADPKD, similar linkage was found with the probes on chromosome 16. It has been suggested that both forms of the disease are due to mutations occurring within the same gene or group of genes. Identification of the gene(s) will provide the answer as to whether the two mutations are actually allelic [9].

In some autosomal dominant diseases, the sex of the carrier has been shown to influence the rate of progression in the offspring. This has so far not been analyzed properly in ADPKD.

Sex. Zeier et al. [1] have suggested that in ADPKD, ESRF occurs later in females than in males, owing to a slower progression of renal failure. In 138 patients (aged 35–65 years) with ESRF due to ADPKD, we found that the mean age at renal death was slightly but not significantly higher in females ($n = 74$) than in males ($n = 64$): 51.7 ± 0.68 vs 50.5 ± 0.14 years (n.s.). The disease did not progress more slowly in females as, among the 90 patients who were followed from the onset of renal failure, females had a slightly but not significantly shorter median renal survival than males. However, we found a striking female preponderance (F/M ratio: 3.7) among 52 patients with slowly progressive ADPKD (17 in whom dialysis was started after age 65, and 35 whose serum creatinine was below 130 μmol/l (at 45–55 years), below 220 μmol/l (at 55–65 years) or at any level over 65 years of age). This may indicate either that this form is more frequent in affected women, or that men with slowly progressive ADPKD are less often detected than females (possibly because urinary tract infection is less prevalent in males).

Hypertension and Other Renal Factors. Hypertension is common in ADPKD patients, it prevalence rising with age [10]. Prominent arteriolar lesions in ADP kidneys suggest that hypertension might play a role in the progression of renal failure in this disease [1], but follow-up studies of ADPKD patients have led to conflicting results. Iglesias et al. [2] have shown that postdiagnosis kidney and patient survivals were better among normotensive ADPKD than among those who were hypertensive at diagnosis. However, mean age at ESRF is not influenced by the presence of hypertension at diagnosis (in our patients) or by the presence of sustained (more than 10 years' duration) hypertension [11]. Moreover, Franz and Reubi [11] found that sustained hypertension also has no influence on the renal deterioration rate. These studies, however, have included relatively small numbers of patients and have not analyzed the potential effect of the various antihypertensive drugs.

Better kidney survival was found in the patients diagnosed from 1956 to 1980 than among those diagnosed between 1935 to 1955 [2]. This may be due to better symptomatic management, including blood pressure control. We have analyzed kidney survival in ADPKD patients who had chronic renal failure (serum creatinine above 200 μmol/l) and who arrived at ESRF either between 1969 and 1975 ($n = 34$) or between 1979 and 1984 ($n = 32$). Median renal survival was slightly higher in the second group than in the first (42 vs 33 months; $p = 0.09$).

It has been suggested that cyst infection and rupture may trigger renal interstitial fibrosis, leading to progressive destruction of the renal parenchyma [1], but no relationship was found between the incidence of upper urinary tract infection and the progression of renal failure [11]. Moreover, progression to renal failure is not faster in affected women [1], in whom upper urinary tract infection is more frequent [12]. Nevertheless, renal infection in ADPKD includes various clinical presentations with various responses to conventional antibiotic therapy [12], whose final consequences on renal function may differ. In women with ADPKD, pregnancy did not appear to exert a deleterious effect on the course of renal disease, and the incidence of pregnancy-induced urinary tract infection was relatively low [13].

Erythrocyte count ranges widely in ADPKD, even in uremic patients. We did not find any relationship between the level of anemia at ESRF and the rate of progression of renal failure.

Extrarenal Manifestations. Familial clustering of intracranial aneurysms has been observed in ADPKD. This association may therefore represent a specific subset [14]. No data is available on DNA linkage analysis or on the rate of renal deterioration in this group of families.

Liver cysts are commonly found in ADPKD. Their prevalence is dependent on patient age: at 60 years or more, approximately 75% of the patients have liver cysts demonstrated by ultrasonography [15]. The expression of the cystic process in the liver is probably hormonally regulated as liver cysts develop earlier and are more voluminous in women than in men. It has been said that the presence of liver cysts is associated with more severe renal involvement [16]. This might only be due to the increased prevalence of liver cysts with age, as we found such lesions in 28 of 37 females (76%) and in 6 of 10 males with slowly progressive ADPKD. The prevalence is the same as in elderly patients with 'classical' ADPKD.

Renal Prognosis in Progressive Hereditary Nephritis

Progressive hereditary nephritis (HN) is a noncystic, nonmetabolic renal disease, characterized by its inherited pattern and its ability to progress to renal failure in the propositus or in the family. Electron microscopy and immunologic studies have pointed to alterations in glomerular basement membrane (GBM) structure and antigenicity. According to the presence or absence of extrarenal involvement (sensorineural hearing loss, lenticonus, perimacular retinal changes), HN has been subdivided into Alport's syndrome (with hearing defect in the family) and HN without deafness (HNWD). Both forms are genetically heterogeneous: the principal mode of inheritance is dominant, most often X-linked, less frequently autosomal; presumed autosomal recessive transmission occurs very rarely [17].

The clinical course of HN is heterogeneous. This has been well documented in women and in men. Women may be asymptomatic carriers with a normal life span, or may progress to ESRF, either early, like males, in some cases, or more often, late, after 50–60 years of age. Affected male patients progress to renal failure in childhood or in adulthood, and some reach ESRF after 50 years of age. Male carriers with no urinary abnormalities have been identified in very rare instances [17]. In order to identify predictive factors, we have recently reanalyzed our data dealing with 129 patients from 39 kindreds with Alport's syndrome and 21 patients from 7 kindreds with HNWD.

Table 1. Median renal survival (years) in hereditary nephritis

	Alport's syndrome		HNWD
	presumed X-linked	autosomal dominant	
Males	25 (n = 56)	51 (n = 20)	34 (n = 10)
Females	57 (n = 47)	not calculated[a] (n = 5)	57 (n = 11)

[a] Two patients were alive with normal renal function at 17 and 42 years, and 3 patients underwent dialysis treatment or died at 58, 70 or 86 years.

Prognostic Factors Related to the Kindred

Atkin et al. [18] indicated that HNWD has a better outcome than Alport's syndrome. In our series, we found no difference in the rate of progression to ESRF in the two groups (table 1). In males, there is a strong correlation between age at renal death in affected relatives [19]. Two groups of families were therefore distinguished, those in which males reach ESRF either before or after 31 years of age [20]. Information regarding prognosis can be drawn from analyzing renal outcome in affected males of the kindred [19]. In contrast, this cannot be done in affected women since there is marked clinical heterogeneity among women in a given family.

The mode of inheritance has some influence on renal prognosis. In our series, median renal survival was higher among the male patients with autosomal dominant Alport's syndrome than in those with X-linked dominant disease (table 1). This can account for the observation that among males, Alport's syndrome inherited from the father carries a better prognosis than Alport's syndrome inherited from the mother [21]. Although we have too few female patients with autosomal dominant Alport's syndrome to perform valid statistical analysis, a similar trend in renal outcome according to the mode of inheritance seems to be present among women (table 1). Such a difference is not surprising since many autosomal dominant diseases (such as ADPKD or Huntington's disease) have delayed appearance of symptoms, contrasting with the earlier clinical presentation of recessive inherited diseases. Obviously, results of DNA studies in the near future will allow more precise analysis of genetic heterogeneity and of gene defects.

Prognostic Factors Related to the Patient

It has long been recognized that renal outcome is poorer in males than in females with Alport's syndrome [17]. In our series (table 1), median renal survival was longer in the 50 affected symptomatic females (61 years) than in the 76 affected males (32 years). A similar difference, although statistical difference was not reached, was found in patients with HNWD. An explanation had been sought in the predominance of X-linked transmission in HN: early random inactivation of one X chromosome in females prevents all of them from fully expressing the defective gene [22]. However, this cannot be the sole explanation since in our study, female sex also carries a good prognosis when analysis was restricted to autosomal dominant Alport's syndrome. As postulated by Brenner [23], androgens may have renotropic effects hastening the course of chronic renal disease, and these effects are possibly involved in other renal diseases, such as IgA, membranous or diabetic nephropathy.

Extrarenal involvement (hearing loss, perimacular changes) carries a poor prognosis in Alport's syndrome [24, 25]. However, since both abnormalities are closely associated with the male sex, their value as independent prognostic factors may be questioned [24, 25]. In our series, we evaluated renal prognosis separately in males and females from 39 kindreds with Alport's syndrome and found no difference in renal survival according to the presence or absence of hearing loss. Heavy proteinuria and the nephrotic syndrome are associated with poor outcome in both sexes [21, 24]. The nephrotic syndrome, usually mild, is observed in approximately 40% of Alport patients, but its incidence is much higher in the kindreds with early progression to renal failure than in those with late progression [17]. In females, gross hematuria in childhood, diffuse thickening of the GBM by electron microscopy and progression of the renal changes by light microscopy on two successive renal biopsies are suggestive of poor prognosis [26]. It should be kept in mind that the absence of significant renal histopathological changes by light microscopy in young children does not preclude further progression to renal failure [17].

References

1 Zeier M, Geberth S, Ritz E, et al: Adult dominant polycystic kidney disease. Clinical problems. Nephron 1988;49:177–183.

2 Iglesias CG, Torres VE, Offord KP, et al: Epidemiology of adult polycystic kidney disease, Olmsted County, Minnesota: 1935-1980. Am J Kidney Dis 1983;2:630–639.

3 Churchill DN, Bear JC, Morgan J, et al: Prognosis of adult onset polycystic kidney disease re-evaluated. Kidney Int 1984;26:190–193.
4 Sedman A, Bell P, Manco-Johnson M. et al: Autosomal dominant polycystic kidney disease in childhood: a longitudinal study. Kidney Int 1987;31:1000–1005.
5 Grantham JJ, Geiser JL, Evan AP: Cyst formation and growth in autosomal dominant polycystic kidney disease. Kidney Int 1987;31:1145–1152.
6 Gabow PA, Ikle DW, Holmes JH: Polycystic kidney disease: prospective analysis of nonazotemic patients and family members. Ann Intern Med 1984;101:238–247.
7 Reeders ST, Breuning MH, Davies KE, et al: A highly polymorphic DNA marker linked to adult polycystic kidney disease on chromosome 16. Nature 1985;317:542–544.
8 Romeo G, Costa G, Catizone L, et al: A second genetic locus for autosomal dominant polycystic kidney disease. Lancet 1988;ii:8–10.
9 Bachner L, Kaplan JC: Molecular genetics and polycystic kidney diseases; in Grünfeld JP, Bach JF, Funck-Brentano JL, Maxwell MH (eds): Advances in Nephrology. Chicago, Year Book, 1988, vol 18.
10 Milutinovic J, Fialkow PJ, Agodoa LY, et al: Autosomal dominant polycystic kidney disease: symptoms and clinical findings. Q J Med 1984;53:511–522.
11 Franz KA, Reubi FC: Rate of functional deterioration in polycystic kidney disease. Kidney Int 1983;23:526–529.
12 Schwab SJ, Bander SJ, Klahr S: Renal infection in autosomal dominant polycystic kidney disease. Am J Med 1987;82:714–718.
13 Jungers P, Forget D, Henry-Amar M, et al: Chronic kidney disease and pregnancy; in Grünfeld JP, Bach JF, Crosnier J, Funck-Brentano, JL, Maxwell MH (eds): Advances in Nephrology. Chicago, Year Book, 1986, vol 15, pp 103–141.
14 Gabow PA, Schrier RW: Pathophysiology of adult polycystic kidney disease: in Grünfeld JP, Bach JF, Funck-Brentano JL, Maxwell MH (eds): Advances in Nephrology. Chicago, Year Book, 1988, vol 18.
15 Grünfeld JP, Albouze G, Jungers P, et al: Liver changes and complications in adult polycystic kidney disease; in Bach JF, Crosnier J, Funck-Brentano JL, Grünfeld JP, Maxwell MH (eds): Advances in Nephrology. Chicago, Year Book, 1985, vol 14, pp 1–20.
16 Milutinovic J, Fialkow PJ, Rudd TC, et al: Liver cysts in patients with autosomal dominant polycystic kidney disease. Am J Med 1980;68:741–744.
17 Gruñfeld JP: The clinical spectrum of hereditary nephritis. Kidney Int 1985;27:83–92.
18 Atkin CL, Gregory MC, Border WA: Alport syndrome; in Schrier RW, Gottschak CW (eds): Strauss and Welt's Diseases of the Kidney, ed 4. Boston, Little Brown, 1986, pp 617–641.
19 Tishler PV, Rosner B: The genetics of the Alport syndrome. Birth Defects 1974; 10:93–99.
20 Hasstedt SJ, Atkin CL, San Juan AC: Genetic heterogeneity among kindreds with Alport syndrome. Am J Hun Genet 1986;38:940–953.
21 Grünfeld JP, Bois EP, Hinglais N: Progressive and nonprogressive hereditary chronic nephritis. Kidney Int 1973;4:216–228.
22 O'Neill WM, Atkin CL, Bloomer HA: Hereditary nephritis: a reexamination of its clinical and genetic features. Ann Intern Med 1978;88:176–182.
23 Brenner BM: Hemodynamically mediated glomerular injury and the progressive nature of kidney disease. Kidney Int 1983;23:647–655.
24 Gubler M, Lévy M, Broyer M, et al: Alport's syndrome. A report of 58 cases and a review of the literature. Am J Med 1981;70:493–505.

25 Perrin D, Jungers P, Grünfeld JP, et al: Perimacular changes in Alport's syndrome. Clin Nephrol 1980;13:163–167.
26 Grünfeld JP, Noël LH, Hafez S, et al: Renal prognosis in women with hereditary nephritis. Clin Nephrol 1985;23:267–271.

Jean-Michel Pochet, MD, Département de Néphrologie, Hôpital Necker,
161 rue de Sèvres, F–75743 Paris Cédex 15 (France)

Oldrizzi L, Maschio G, Rugiu C, et al. (eds): The Progressive Nature of Renal Disease: Myths and Facts. Contrib Nephrol. Basel, Karger, 1989, vol 75, pp 108–116

The Natural History of Hypertensive Vascular Nephropathy

Alba Vangelista, Andrea Buscaroli, Claudio Campieri, Vittorio Bonomini

Institute of Nephrology, St. Orsola University Hospital, Bologna, Italy

Hypertensive vascular nephropathy may be defined as the renal function and morphological damage caused by arterial hypertension. Since the kidney may be either the target organ or the cause of hypertension, the natural history of hypertensive vascular nephropathy may only be studied in essential hypertension, a condition where the rise in blood pressure is the first demonstrable alteration in the patient, any damage to organs being secondary to hypertension.

The range of renal lesions associated with arterial hypertension is generally encompassed by the term 'nephrosclerosis', which has been further differentiated into 'benign' and 'malignant' nephrosclerosis according to the type and degree of vascular damage. The terms benign and malignant were first used, from the clinical and pathological point of view, by Volhard and Fahr [1] to differentiate the two phases of essential hypertension. Bed-side and desk-side experience has progressively helped to modify this original classification, and today four phases are recognized in essential hypertension: (1) mild; (2) moderate; (3) severe; (4) malignant. Each has its own clinical signs, alterations in renal function, and renal parenchymal changes, and these, though not always equivalent in severity, are all present at one and the same time. It may be argued that the more severe the hypertension, and the longer it is present, the more severe is the histopathology in the kidney and the impact on renal function [2].

Frequency

Among the 14,096 patients admitted to our Nephrological Department in the last 10 years, hypertension was present in 33% of patients, and essential hypertension in 14% of all hypertensives. In morphological terms, a vascular nephropathy was diagnosed in 15% of the 7,144 renal biopsies performed from 1957 to the end of 1987. Essential hypertension represented 74% of vascular nephropathies.

The use of renal biopsy has been of decisive importance in clarifying the natural history of hypertensive vascular nephropathy. Systematic use of biopsy dates from 1943 with surgical biopsies performed during sympathectomy in order to evaluate the frequency and characteristics of arteriolar lesions in hypertensive patients [3]; but only after the contribution of Heptinstall [4] did the importance of renal biopsy become evident in diagnosing the causes of arterial hypertension, and the information so far achieved has progressively reduced the need for biopsy in this condition. Investigations on renal biopsy and autopsy material showed that vascular lesions in the kidney are present in 93–100% of hypertensive patients, as compared to 12% of subjects with normal blood pressure [5].

Phases of Evolution

It is difficult to establish when renal alterations take place in the early course of essential hypertension; the behavior of blood pressure may vary remarkably from patient to patient; the various phases of hypertension may cover different periods of time; sometimes the mild or moderate phases persist for many years; sometimes the passage to the malignant phase occurs rapidly a few months after the onset of hypertension. Essential hypertension, in fact, may be a relatively nonprogressive condition in certain individuals, but in others, even with the same blood pressure levels, there may be more evidence of vascular disease occurring at an earlier stage, and more intensively [6]. Apart from the malignant phase, where renal failure develops in most patients, a definite renal insufficiency has been documented in 4.5–23% of the hypertensive population [7]. Evidence of nephrosclerosis, however, has been observed in most patients with untreated hypertension lasting for more than 5 years [2].

In the *first phase (mild)* of essential hypertension the rise in blood pressure is unstable. Studies on renal hemodynamics show an increase in renal blood flow (RBF) and glomerular filtration rate (GFR), associated with a greater natriuresis after salt load than in normal subjects [8].

Renal vascular lesions are characterized by focal hyaline changes, consisting of irregular deposition of hyaline material along the vascular wall, mostly affecting the afferent arterioles (fig. 1a). Glomeruli are generally normal.

In *phase 2 (moderate)* hypertension is stable, but diastolic blood pressure (DBP) does not exceed 110 mm Hg. The earliest renal function abnormality seems to be a reduction in tubular function (Tm_{PAI}). There is

a b c d

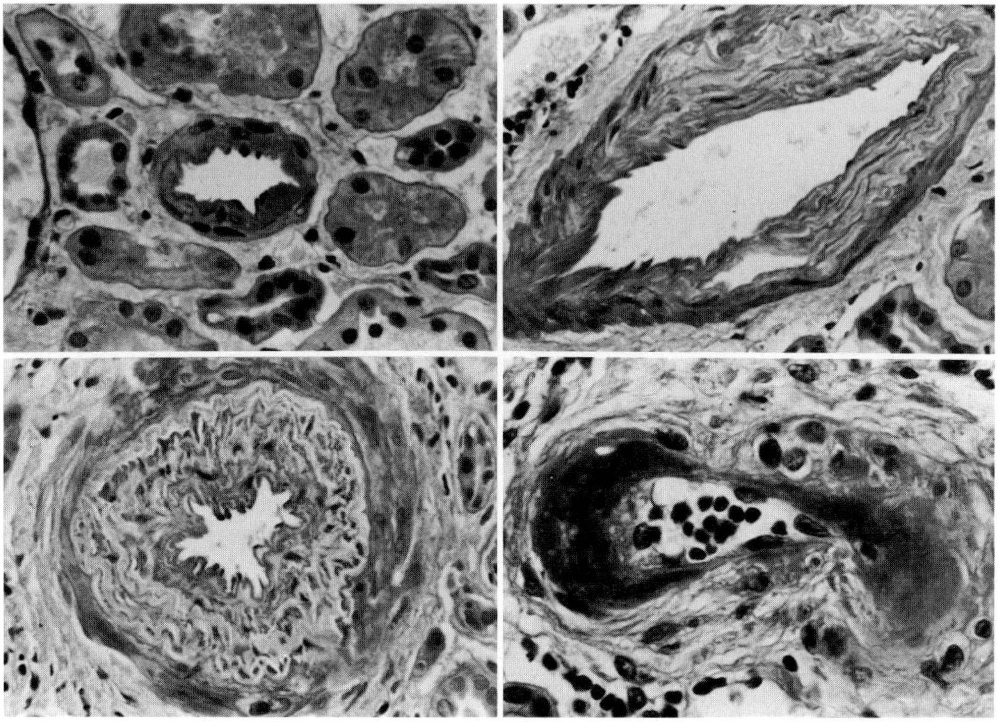

Fig. 1. Renal vascular damage in essential hypertension. *a* Mild hypertension; a preglomerular arteriola with segmental hyalinization of the wall. PAS. × 230. *b* Moderate hypertension; an interlobular arteria with thickening of the wall. The lumen diameter is not reduced. PAS. × 230. *c* Severe hypertension; remarkable thickening of the wall of an interlobular arteria with reduplication of the internal elastic lamina. The vessel's lumen is remarkably reduced. *d* Malignant hypertension; fibrinoid necrosis of the wall of an afferent arteriola. PAS. × 350.

a certain decrease in RBF, while GFR is generally normal, so filtration fraction is increased [7].

Renal vascular lesions are characterized by the extension of hyalinization to the entire arteriolar wall. The interlobular arteries show medial hypertrophy and fibrosis (fig. 1b), but the luminal diameter is still maintained. Glomeruli may show focal ischemic changes characterized by thickening and wrinkling of capillary walls, and tuft shrinkage. There may be focal tubular atrophy with thickening and splitting of the tubular basement membrane and some intraluminal casts.

In *phase 3 (severe)* there is a marked increase in DBP. RBF continues to decrease. GFR is at first maintained by an increase in efferent arteriolar tone in order to preserve glomerular hydrostatic pressure; then a decline takes place, sometimes with a progression to renal insufficiency. The development of terminal renal failure, however, is uncommon in the absence of an accelerated malignant phase [9]. Other manifestations of severe hypertension include decreased tubular concentrating ability, and mild proteinuria.

Renal vascular lesions are characterized by a remarkable thickening of the walls of interlobular arteries and arterioles, fraying and reduplication of the internal elastic lamina, and intimal thickening. The luminal diameter is reduced (fig. 1c). Glomeruli show varying degrees of ischemic changes up to sclerosis. Totally sclerosed glomeruli may be intermingled with normal or hypertrophied glomeruli. Tubulo-interstitial lesions include tubular atrophy and loss, and interstitial fibrosis with or without inflammatory cells.

The *malignant phase* of hypertension may develop after one to 30 years of benign hypertension, but sometimes it occurs suddenly in patients with no previous history of hypertension. DBP is usually greater than 130 mm Hg. The major clinical features include neurological abnormalities, severe headache, weight loss, and diagnostic funduscopic alterations characterized by papilledema, hemorrage and exudates. In most cases renal failure develops rapidly, and in untreated patients it accounts for over two thirds of deaths during the first year from the onset. The incidence of malignant hypertension in the hypertensive population has been reported to vary from 1% [9] to7% [10]. Its frequency has progressively reduced with time, very probably because of earlier diagnosis and more appropriate treatment of hypertension.

In the kidney the hallmark of malignant hypertension is fibrinoid necrosis of arteriolar walls (fig. 1d). Mural hemorrhage and thrombosis may also be present. A second vascular change which occurs in malignant hypertension is proliferative endoarteritis, characterized by a marked endothelial proliferation with pseudoelastic fiber formation in a concentric fashion affecting the afferent arterioles and interlobular arteries (onion-skin appearance), and resulting in a remarkable narrowing of the lumen. Glomerular lesions may be variable according to whether the malignant phase is superimposed on a longstanding hypertension, or whether it occurs primarily. The most impressive change is the fibrinoid necrosis which may affect the entire capillary tuft, but more often involves only a portion. The cells lining the Bowman's capsule may proliferate, and the capillaries may be blood filled. The number of glomeruli affected may vary from 5 to 30% [11].

Clinicopathological Correlations

In order to define the relationship between the clinical phase of essential hypertension and the degree of functional and pathological renal

Table 1. Hypertensive patients in whom a renal biopsy had been performed, grouped according to the phase of essential hypertension

Phases of hypertension	Patients
I Mild	15
II Moderate	28
III Severe	43
IV Malignant	19
	105

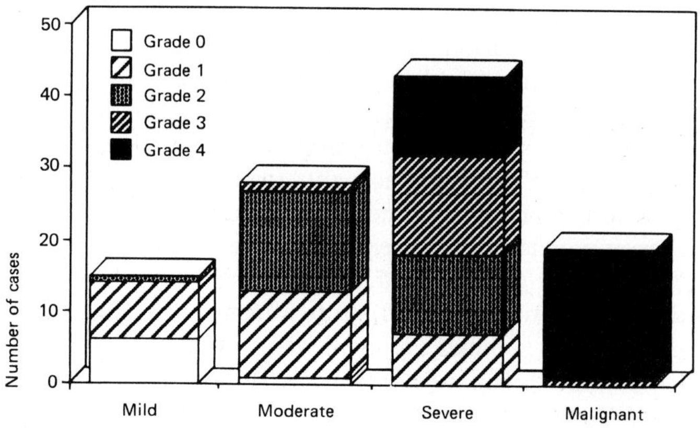

Fig. 2. Degree of renal arteriolar damage observed at renal biopsy in 105 patients with essential hypertension, grouped according to the phase of hypertension. PAS. × 400.

damage, we analyzed the renal biopsy specimens of 105 patients studied in different phases of the hypertensive disease (table 1). Only patients under the age of 60 years have been included, to avoid the presence of age-related vascular changes in the kidney. Hypertension duration ranged from 3 months to 15 years. A severe vascular damage was mainly found in phases 3 and 4 (fig. 2). There was a good correlation between the severity of DBP and the degree of both arteriolar damage (fig. 3a) and glomerular sclerosis (fig. 3b). In terms of renal function, no correlation was found between hypertension duration and serum creatinine at the time of renal biopsy. On the contrary, the latter significantly correlated with the height of DBP (fig. 3c) and the degree of vascular damage in the kidney (fig. 3d).

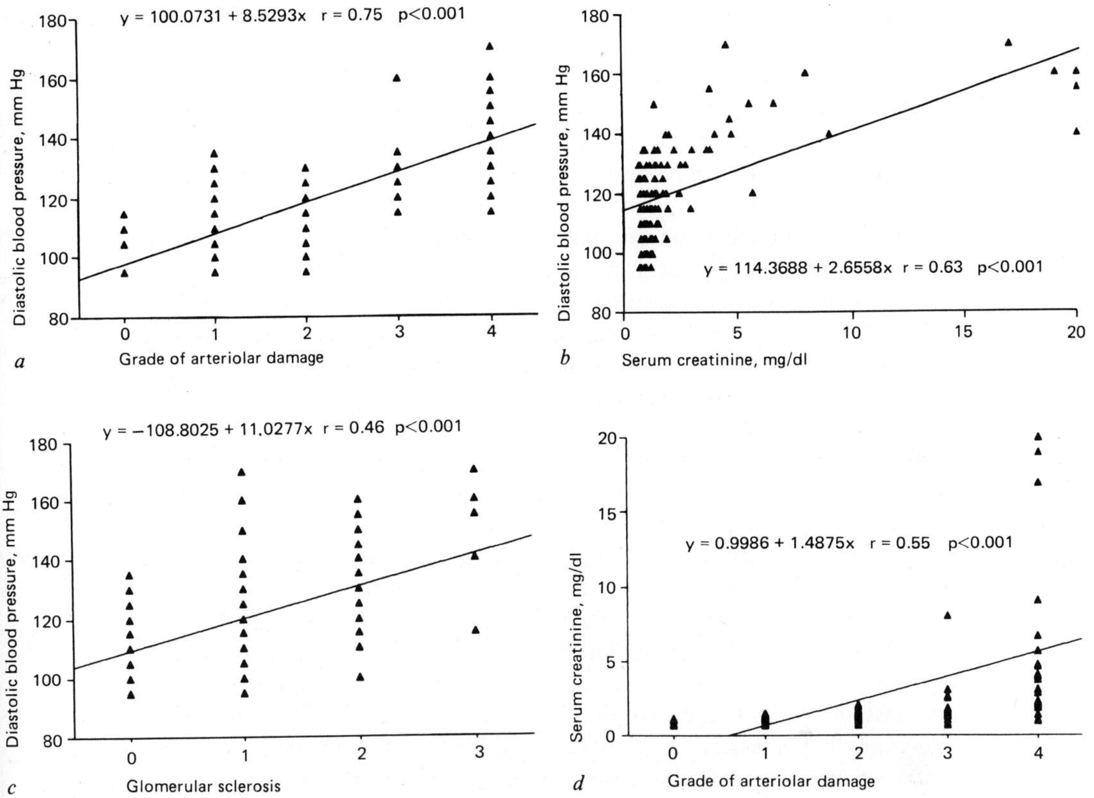

Fig. 3. Clinicopathological correlations in 105 patients with essential hypertension. *a* Correlation between the height of diastolic blood pressure and the degree of arteriolar lesions in the kidney. *b* Correlation between the height of diastolic blood pressure and the degree of glomerular sclerosis in the kidney. *c* Correlation between the height of diastolic blood pressure and serum creatinine at the time of renal biopsy. *d* Correlation between serum creatinine at the time of renal biopsy and the degree of arteriola lesions in the kidney.

Mechanisms of Progression

The progression of renal vascular lesions in essential hypertension can be summarized as follows: (1) irregular deposition of hyaline material in the arteriolar wall; (2) extension of hyalinization and replacement by sclerotic tissue; (3) thickening of the wall of interlobular arteries and arterioles with elastic reduplication and lumen reduction; (4) onion-skin appearance and fibrinoid necrosis. The sequence of these evolutional stages can take place over a few to many years of hypertension. Sometimes the onset of malignant hypertension may be the first clinical manifestation of the disease. The renal changes of hypertensive disease may be halted, reversed or prevented by an adequate control of systemic blood pressure.

When the hypertensive disease progresses, the kidney not only undergoes more and more severe damage as target organ, but in turn it becomes responsible for the progression of hypertensive disease. The mutual influence between systemic hypertension and renal function is typical: reciprocal coexistence and adaptation for even long periods of time; a rapid worsening in both when either of them disturb the balance. In hypertensive vascular nephropathy it is usually the blood pressure which first breaks this balance. In other chronic nephropathies, the worsening in renal function precedes the rise in blood pressure. This is not a constant rule, but it has to be mentioned because of its clinical implications.

There is no doubt that among the risk factors which lead to the progression of renal damage, inadequate antihypertensive treatment is the most important, whether through use of inadequate drugs, inadequate use of appropriate drugs, or failure of the patient to comply with treatment. For example, the frequent use and overuse of diuretics may play a role in worsening the hypertension, especially in its advanced stage. In this condition the reduced adaptability of renal hemodynamics makes more evident the effects of the RAS stimulation associated with the diuretic-induced volume depletion. Some investigators have suggested that the RAS may be involved in the pathogenesis of the fibrinoid arteriolar lesions found in malignant hypertension. It is well recognized that renin and angiotensin blood levels are usually increased in this condition. Renin administration can produce vascular changes similar to those found in malignant hypertension [12]. Moreover the lack of a demonstration of a high renin activity in peripheral blood does not exclude a relative stimulation of the RAS in the kidney. This might be responsible for the imbalance between afferent and efferent arteriolar resistances, and the glomerular capillary hypertension which follows, and leads to a more rapid progression of renal structural and functional damage [13].

Plans for Therapy

In the initial phases of essential hypertension the control of blood pressure by means of antihypertensive drugs is crucial if the onset of hypertensive vascular damage is to be prevented. When renal vascular lesions have already taken place, there may be the transition to the 'RAS phase', which may be triggered by the inadequate control of blood pressure and/or by the excessive use of diuretics. Local RAS stimulation, in fact, may be induced by both baroreceptor and chemoreceptor mechanisms. Antihypertensive therapy with ACE inhibitors and calcium antagonists may be effective in this condition, even in the absence of any increase in peripheral renin activity. It has also been demonstrated that the renal effects of ACE inhibitors are better than those achievable with other antihypertensive drugs, despite a similar control of blood pressure [14]. In patients with malignant hypertension associated with renal insufficiency, vigorous antihypertensive treatment may results in renal function improvement in 60% of patients, with an overall one-year patient survival rate of 69% [15].

When hypertension persists, the renal consequence is nephroangiosclerosis; the extrarenal consequence is represented by generalized vascular damage (i.e. atherosclerosis, whether accelerated or not). When renal failure takes place, early substitution therapy with dialysis or transplantation represents the most effective approach in order to reduce the progression of accelerated atherosclerosis [16]. It is the only approach which may improve patient survival in the uremic phase of hypertensive vascular nephropathy, up to the levels of other chronic nephropathies, of glomerular or tubulo-interstitial origin.

References

1 Volahrd F, Fahr T: Die Brightsche Nierekrankheit: Klinik, Pathologie und Atlas. Berlin, Springer, 1914.

2 Lindeman RD, Tobin JD, Shock NW: Hypertension and the kidney. Nephron 1987;47(suppl 1):62–67.

3 Castleman B, Smithwick RH: The relation of vascular disease to the hypertensive state. JAMA 1943;121:1256–1261.

4 Heptinstall RH: Renal biopsies in hypertension. Br Heart J 1954;16:133–141.

5 Samarq P: La biopsie rénale dans l'hypertension artérielle dite essentielle; in Actualités Néphrologiques de l'Hopital Necker. Paris, Flammarion, 1961, pp 215–222.

6 Edwards JC: Management of Hypertensive Disease. St. Louis, Mosby, 1960, pp 86–102.

7 Schwartz GL, Strong CG: Renal parenchymal involvement in essential hypertension. Med Clin North Am 1987;71:843–858.

8 Bianchi G, Cusi D, Guidi E: Renal hemodynamics in human subjects and in animals with genetic hypertension during the prehypertensive stage. Am J Nephrol 1983;3:73–79.

9 Kincaid-Smith P: The Kidney. A Clinico-Pathological Study. Oxford, Blackwell, 1975, p 205.

10 Perera GA: Hypertensive vascular disease: description and natural history. J Chronic Dis 1955;1:33–42.

11 Heptinstall RH: Pathology of the Kidney. Boston, Little, Brown, 1974, p 121.

12 Humpreys MH, Alfrey AC: Vascular diseases of the kidney; in Brenner BM, Rector FC (eds): The Kidney. Philadelphia, Saunders, 1986, pp 1175–1220.

13 Anderson G, Meyer TW, Rennke HG, Brenner BM: Control of glomerular hypertension limits glomerular injury in rats with reduced renal mass. J Clin Invest 1985;76:612–619.
14 Ledingham JGG: Severe hypertension. Is there a drug of choice? Nephron 1987;47(suppl 1):47–50.
15 Lawton WJ: The short-term course of renal function in malignant hypertension with renal insufficiency. Clin Nephrol 1982;6:277–283.
16 Bonomini V, Feletti C, Scolari MP, Stefoni S, Vangelista A: Atherosclerosis in uremia: a longitudinal study. Am J Clin Nutr 1980;33:1493–1500.

Prof. Vittorio Bonomini, Cattedra di Nefrologia Medica, Ospedale Sant Orsola, Via Massarenti 9, I–40138 Bologna (Italy)

Oldrizzi L, Maschio G, Rugiu C, et al. (eds): The Progressive Nature of Renal Disease: Myths and Facts. Contrib Nephrol. Basel, Karger, 1989, vol 75, pp 117–126

Natural History and Treatment of Diabetic Nephropathy

G. C. Viberti

Unit for Metabolic Medicine, UMDS, Guy's Campus, London, England, UK

Diabetic kidney disease becomes clinically overt in approximately 35% of patients with insulin-dependent diabetes mellitus [1, 2] and in an ill-defined but supposedly smaller proportion of about 10% of patients of European origin with non-insulin-dependent diabetes mellitus. Large ethnic variations are seen in the incidence of diabetic kidney disease in non-insulin-dependent diabetic patients and a higher incidence is found in those populations who develop the disease at an earlier age such as the Japanese, Asian and American Indians, and Mexicans. In these ethnic groups, some of whom also afford some protection from coronary heart disease, more 'diabetes time' is available for the renal disease to manifest itself. Diabetic kidney disease accounts for much of the premature mortality of diabetic patients [3] and is rapidly becoming the single most common cause of end-stage renal failure. In some countries, diabetic patients represent up to one third of all patients receiving renal replacement treatment [4, 5].

Overt Diabetic Kidney Disease

Diabetic nephropathy is characterised by persistent proteinuria (i.e. total urinary protein > 0.5 g/24 h), arterial hypertension, declining glomerular filtration rate (GFR) and plasma lipid abnormalities. The disease, under ordinary circumstances, progresses relentlessly, and premature mortality occurs from uraemia and, in about a third of cases, cardiovascular disease [3]. With the appearance of persistent proteinuria, a decline of GFR is inexorably established at rates varying between 0.5 and 2.4 ml/min/month in different individuals [6]. Arterial pressure starts to climb at a very early stage of renal involvement in diabetes, and different degrees of rise and control seem to influence the speed of GFR fall [7, 8]. With the decline of GFR, proteinuria and the clearance of major plasma proteins such as

Table 1. Effect of low protein intake on the rate of GFR decline and total urinary protein excretion in 19 clinically proteinuric, insulin-dependent diabetic patients. Data are mean $\pm$ SEM.

	Normal protein diet	Low-protein diet	Significance level
Total urinary protein, g/24 h	2.9 ± 0.4	1.5 ± 0.4	$p < 0.01$
GFR fall, ml/min/month	0.7 ± 0.1	0.2 ± 0.1	$p < 0.02$
Glycosylated Hb, %	9.2 ± 0.4	9.4 ± 0.6	n.s.

albumin and IgG increase. There is a change from a proteinuria highly selective for albumin in the early stages, when the GFR is normal or only moderately reduced, to a low selectivity proteinuria with proportionally more IgG being cleared when the GFR is markedly reduced [9].

Increases in LDL and VLDL cholesterol and triglyceride, as well as decreases in HDL_2 cholesterol, accompany the progression of the disease [10, 11]. Prevailing levels of glycaemic control seem to be little related to the progression of renal failure once it has entered this advanced phase [12, 13]. The relationship between arterial pressure and the deterioration of renal function seems closest at this stage. In a carefully followed series, vigorous treatment of raised blood pressure lowered the rate of decline of GFR from 0.9 ml/min/month before treatment to 0.2 ml/min/month treatment. This lower rate of fall was maintained for several years and concomitantly albuminuria was reduced, though not entirely normalised [8]. The anti-hypertensive regimen used in these early studies included selective β-blockers, vasodilators and diuretics. More recently a number of studies, though uncontrolled and small in size, seem to suggest that the administration of angiotensin converting enzyme inhibitors to diabetic renal failure patients may have additional beneficial effects on the progression of renal disease. Some workers have claimed that these results are independent of systemic blood pressure reduction, and animal studies suggest that they may be related to the lowering of intraglomerular pressure [14–16].

Therapeutic manoeuvres likely to affect glomerular haemodynamics are therefore likely to be beneficial; in this respect, restriction of dietary protein intake may prove useful. Persistently proteinuric, insulin-dependent diabetic patients aged between 30 and 64 years with a mean duration of diabetes of 24 years were studied over a period of at least 4 years, the last two of which on restricted protein intake. The prescribed low-protein diet reduced protein intake from 81 ± 21 to 46 ± 6 g/day. This manoeuvre was accompanied by a significant fall in total protein excretion and rate of decline of GFR (table 1). Moreover, the low-protein diet also reduced the elevated serum levels of cholesterol and LDL cholesterol present in these patients. Even though the response to a low-protein diet was heterogenous, with some individuals markedly slowing their rate of progression and others showing little change, these findings support the view that, on average, a low-protein diet has a beneficial and independent effect on the evolution of renal failure and may correct some of the attendant lipid disturbances [17, 18]. The mechanisms by which reduction of dietary protein affect progression of diabetic renal disease in man are not entirely clear. Short-term low-protein intake reduces proteinuria but does not alter baseline renal haemodynamics, nor does it restore to physiologic levels the impaired renal vasodilatory response to protein intake [19, 20]. Further controlled studies are needed to substantiate the promising results obtained with reduction of blood pressure and dietary protein intake, but the available evidence suggests that progression of overt diabetic nephropathy can not be significantly retarded. However no intervention to date has been able to arrest or reverse this condition. By the time the clinical diagnosis is made, the renal lesions may be too far advanced and irreversible by present therapeutic means. Early identification of patients at risk of developing diabetic nephropathy becomes therefore important.

Early Renal Changes

A proportion of approximately 20% of non-proteinuric insulin-dependent diabetic patients excrete albumin at rates well above normal but below the detection limit of usual routine tests. These subclinical elevations of albumin excretion fall between 30 and 300 mg/24 h and are defined as microalbuminuria. Prospective studies have demonstrated that diabetic patients with microalbuminuria have a 20-fold higher risk of developing clinical nephropathy [21] and in the non-insulin-dependent patients a greater risk of early cardiovascular mortality [22, 23].

Recent findings indicate that levels of albumin excretion rate identifying at-risk patients are absent during the first 5 years of diabetes in conventionally treated, insulin-dependent diabetic patients [24]; this suggests that microalbuminuria is a sign of early disease rather than a marker of susceptibility to it. Different studies have shown that microalbuminuria is associated with poor glycaemic control and, perhaps more importantly, is related independently and more closely with raised levels of arterial pressure [25, 26]. By and large microalbuminuric diabetic patients have arterial pressures within conventionally accepted non-hypertensive levels, but the values are significantly higher than those expected for their age (table 2). Thus, the association between raised arterial pressure and

Table 2. Arterial pressure in age-, sex- and duration-matched, insulin-dependent diabetic patients with albumin excretion rates (AER) above (n = 12) and below 30 μg/min (n = 28). Data are mean ± SEM

	AER	
	above 30 μg/min	below 30 μg/min
Systolic BP, mm Hg	136 ± 5	118 ± 2**
Diastolic BP, mm Hg	87 ± 3	76 ± 2*

*p < 0.005; **p < 0.005.

proteinuria is present well before the stage of overt nephropathy and it occurs in the absence of any renal hypofunction, GFR being either normal or elevated at this stage. Concomitant with these changes is the presence of left ventricular hypertrophy in microalbuminuric diabetic patients [27]. It is unclear at present whether the higher blood pressures are the result of existing kidney disease, though subclinical, or whether it is those diabetic patients with blood pressures in the upper reaches of the normal distribution who are more likely to develop microalbuminuria, thus initiating the vicious circle of hypertension and kidney disease characteristic of late nephropathy. Another association of microalbuminuria with potentially important prognostic implications is that with higher levels of plasma lipids as recently shown is a case control study [28]. Thus, diabetic patients at the stage of microalbuminuria already display all the features that characteristically increase the risk of renal and cardiovascular complications.

Other early physiological renal abnormalities occur in diabetes. Supranormal values of GFR can be found in diabetic patients. Cross-sectionally, an elevated GFR can be associated with either normal of subclinically elevated levels of albumin excretion and, vice versa, microalbuminuria may be accompanied by a high or normal GFR [29]. Whether there is a chronological relationship between increases in GFR and in albumin excretion rate, with the former preceding the latter, remains to be established in man. In experimental diabetic animals, elevated GFR has been implicated in the initiation and progression of diabetic renal disease [16], but this has not yet been proven in humans. A small selected group of hyperfiltering diabetic patients, in whom the high GFR was coupled with microalbuminuria, was found to progress to persistent proteinuria and lose glomerular function, over a 10-year period, at a significantly higher rate than a control group with lower GFR and normal albumin excretion rate

Table 3. GFR and AER in 10 healthy subjects on animal or vegetable protein diets containing equivalent amount of protein (~ 80 g/day)

	Animal protein diet	Vegetable protein diet
GFR, ml/min/1.73 m^2	121 ± 4	110 ± 4**
AER, μg/min	11.2 ± 1.9	4.9 ± 0.6*

*p < 0.02; **p < 0.006.

[30]. This study cannot dissect out the independent contribution of glomerular hyperfiltration to the progression of renal damage but is compatible with the view that an elevation of the GFR may play a role in the sequence of events leading to diabetic renal failure.

Treatment of Early Renal and Systemic Pressure Abnormalities

The early phase changes respond to a number of therapeutic manoeuvres. Intensified insulin treatment and strict glycaemic control can correct glomerular hyperfiltration and microalbuminuria or, at worst, prevent the progressive rise of albumin excretion rate in at-risk individuals [31, 32].

Correction of the marginal elevations of arterial pressure by angiotensin-converting enzyme inhibitors as well as by diuretic or selective β-blockers also reduces microalbuminuria [33, 34]. Short-term studies of restriction of dietary protein intake has shown that a diet containing approximately 45 g of protein daily is capable of reducing both microalbuminuria and GFR independently of blood glucose and arterial pressure changes [35]. The reduction in albumin excretion rate exceeded that of the GFR, leading to significant fall in the fractional clearance of albumin, suggesting an amelioration of the permselectivity properties of the glomerular barrier. Recent observations in healthy humans with different protein intake indicate that vegans who eat less protein, all of which is vegetable in origin, have significantly lower GFR, albumin excretion rates and arterial pressures than those of omnivorous subjects who eat more protein, largely of animal origin [36]. Moreover when omnivorous individuals are fed a vegan diet containing the same amount of protein, both GFR and urinary albumin excretion decrease significantly (table 3). For equivalent protein content a vegan diet therefore seems to be associated with renal changes that should confer protection against nephropathy in diabetes.

Thus, effective measures of post-primary prevention are available, and though many of the mechanisms by which lowering of blood pressure and restriction or modification of protein intake operate are still obscure, it is of great relevance that their effect is independent of glycaemic control.

Only long-term controlled trials will reveal whether correction of an early indicator of disease leads to abolition of the disease itself. The question remains as to whether patients susceptible to diabetic nephropathy could be identified at diagnosis of diabetes by some marker, probably genetic, present well before microalbuminuria or other risk indicators appear.

Blood Pressure and Susceptibility to Nephropathy

It is clear that only a minority, albeit a large one, of diabetic patients develops renal failure [1, 2]. Although this is partly explained by the quality of metabolic control, other factors appear to be equally important. The finding that elevation of arterial pressure is present in microalbuminuric diabetic patients without renal hypofunction, and that long-term uncomplicated diabetic survivors have low arterial pressures [37], suggests that the relationship between hypertension and diabetic renal disease is more complex than previously believed. Although rises in arterial pressure are generally considered the consequence of the renal disease, other interpretations are possible. It is possible that increases in blood pressure play a contributory role in the pathogenesis of diabetic renal disease or that hypertension and renal damage are the manifestations of a common disturbed mechanism. A familial predisposition to raised arterial pressure may be a factor that contributes to the susceptibility to nephropathy, when diabetes is present. This hypothesis is supported by the finding that parents of proteinuric diabetic patients have significantly higher arterial pressure level than age and body mass index matched parents of non-proteinuric diabetics [38].

A significant correlation is found between arterial pressures in the proteinuric diabetic patients and those in their respective parents. These data have been complemented by the finding that rates of red cell sodium-lithium counter-transport, a system the activity of which is associated with the risk of essential hypertension, are higher in proteinuric and microalbuminuric diabetic patients than in watched, long-term normoalbuminuric patients [39, 40]. The risk of nephropathy seems to be magnified by the combination of a previous history of poor glycaemic control and the possession of a high sodium-lithium counter-transport activity [40].

It is believed that the activity of sodium-lithium counter-transport closely relates to that of the physiologic sodium-hydrogen antiport. This

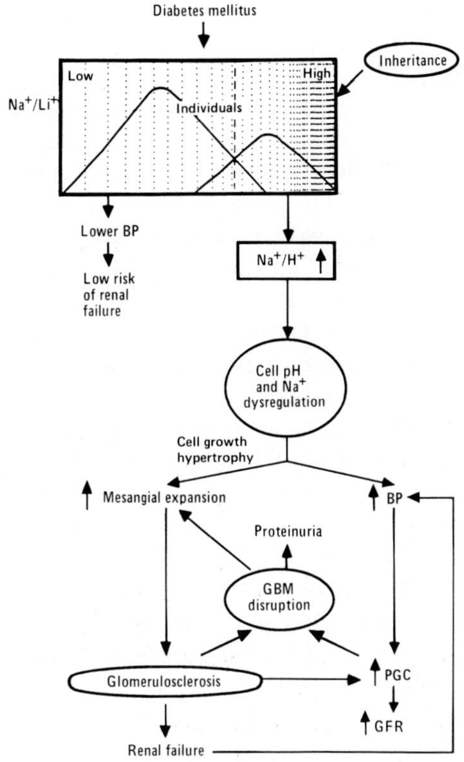

Fig. 1. Diagrammatic representation of a hypothetical sequence of events leading to diabetic renal failure. The graph in the rectangular box represents the bimodal distribution of sodium-lithium counter-transport activity (Na^+/Li^+) in the general population. High values averaging 0.55 mmol/l RBC/h are present in about 13% of the population. The stippled area represents the level of diabetic control. The denser dots indicate the worse control. It is assumed that the level of sodium-lithium counter-transport activity reflects the activity of the sodium-hydrogen (Na^+/H^+) antiport. It is postulated that the combination of poorly controlled diabetes with an inherited predisposition to higher levels of Na^+/H^+ exchanger activity would lead to chronic overactivation of the antiport. The sequence of events that would follow is illustrated and commented on in detail in the text.

system is crucial in the control of intracellular pH, and therefore cell growth, and in the renal proximal tubule, of sodium reabsorption. Thus, when diabetes occurs in an individual with abnormalities in the sodium-hydrogen counter-transport activity a certain sequence of events may take place. In susceptible individuals with an inherited predisposition to supra-normal activity of sodium-hydrogen counter-transport the environmental changes induced by poorly controlled diabetes may lead, through chronic overactivation of the sodium-hydrogen antiport, to significant dysregulation of intracellular pH and sodium. An increase in intracellular pH may lead to cell hypertrophy and hyperplasia and contribute in the kidney to glomerular hypertrophy and mesangial expansion as well as tubular hypertrophy and hyperplasia. An increased sodium reabsorption by the tubular brush border membrane would augment systemic and renal perfusion pressure to maintain sodium balance. The increased perfusion pressure would be readily transmitted to the glomerular capillaries because of the general vasodilation present in diabetes. This would lead to increased intraglomerular pressure which determines, at least in part, the increase in GFR and may be responsible for the disruption of the glomerular membrane permeability properties contributing to proteinuria. On the other hand progressive mesangial expansion would lead to glomerulosclerosis and further disruption of glomerular basement membrane permselectivity properties. This sequence of phenomena would trigger a vicious circle of events leading to reduction in renal function, more hypertension, more proteinuria, more severe glomerulosclerosis and finally glomerular obsolescence and renal failure. Figure 1 diagrammatically describes the hypothetical steps leading susceptible diabetic individuals to end-stage renal disease. In this scheme poor glycaemic control and an intrinsic cell membrane abnormalities of the Na^+/H^+ antiport in the kidney, would predispose to systemic hypertension and diabetic renal damage.

References

1 Andersen AR, Sandahl Christiansen J, Andersen JK, et al: Diabetic nephropathy in type 1 (insulin-dependent) diabetes. An epidemiological study. Diabetologia 1983;25:496–501.

2 Krolewski AS, Warram JH, Christlieb AR, et al: The changing natural history of nephropathy in type 1 diabetes. Am J Med 1985;78:785–794.

3 Borch-Johnsen K, Andersen PK, Deckert T: The effect on relative mortality in type I (insulin-dependent) diabetes mellitus. Diabetologia 1985;28:251–262.

4 Cameron JS, Challah S: Treatment of end stage renal failure due to diabetes in the United Kingdom 1975–1984. Lancet 1986;ii:962–966.

5 Khanna R, Wu G, Chisholm L, et al: Further experiences with CAPD in diabetics with end-stage renal disease. Diabetic Nephropathy 1983;2:8–12.

6 Viberti GC, Bilous RW, Mackintosh D, et al: Monitoring glomerular function in diabetic nephropathy. A prospective study. Am J Med 1983;74:256–263.

7 Mogensen CE: Progression of nephropathy in long-term diabetics with proteinuria and effects of initial antihypertensive treatment. Scand J Clin Lab Invest 1976;36:383–388.

8 Parving HH, Andersen AR, Smidt UM, et al: Effect of antihypertensive treatment on kidney function in diabetic nephropathy. Br Med J 1987;294:1443–1447.

9 Viberti GC, Keen H: The patterns of proteinuria in diabetes mellitus. Diabetes 1987;36:556–565.

10 Vannini P, Ciavarella A, Flammini M, et al: Lipid abnormalities in insulin-dependent diabetic patients with albuminuria. Diabetes Care 1984;7:151–154.
11 Jensen T, Stender S, Deckert T: Abnormalities in plasma concentrations of lipoprotein and fibrinogen in type 1 (insulin-dependent) diabetic patients with increased urinary albumin excretion. Diabetologia 1988;31:142–145.
12 Viberti GC, Bilous RW, Mackintosh D, et al: Long-term correction of hyperglycaemia and progression of renal failure in insulin-dependent diabetes. Br Med J 1983;286:598–602.
13 Viberti GC, Keen H, Dodds R, et al: Metabolic control and progression of diabetic nephropathy. Diabetologia 1987;30:481–482.
14 Taguma Y, Kitamoto Y, Futaki G, et al: Effect of captopril on heavy proteinuria in azotemic diabetics. N Engl J Med 1985;313:1617–1620.
15 Bjorck S, Nyberg G, Mulec H, et al: Beneficial effects of angiotensin converting enzyme inhibition on renal function in patients with nephropathy. Br Med J 1986;293:471–474.
16 Zatz R, Meyer TW, Rennke HG, et al: Predominance of haemodynamic rather than metabolic factors in the pathogenesis of diabetic glomerulopathy. Proc Natl Acad Sci USA 1985;82:5936–5967.
17 Bending JJ, Dodds RJ, Walker JD, et al: Dietary protein restriction delays the progression of diabetic renal failure. Diabetologia 1987;30:498A.
18 Walker J, Mattock M, Dodds R, et al: Dietary protein restriction modifies lipoprotein abnormalities in insulin-dependent diabetics with nephropathy. Kidney Int 1988;33:213.
19 Bending JJ, Dodds R, Keen H, et al: Renal response to restricted protein intake in diabetic nephropathy. Diabetes, in press.
20 Pinto JR, Bending JJ, Dodds R, et al: Failure of low-protein diet to remove the physiological response to protein ingestion in proteinuric type 1 (insulin-dependent) diabetic patients. Diabetologia 1988;31:531A.
21 Viberti GC, Hill RD, Jarrett RD, et al: Microalbuminuria as a predictor of clinical nephropathy in insulin-dependent diabetes mellitus. Lancet 1982;i:1430–1432.
22 Jarrett RJ, Viberti GC, Argyropoulos A, et al: Microalbuminuria predicts mortality in non-insulin-dependent diabetics. Diabetes Med 1984;1:17–19.
23 Mogensen CE: Mircroalbuminuria predicts clinical proteinuria and early mortality in maturity-onset diabetes. N Engl Med 1984;310:356–360.
24 Close CF: On behalf of the MCS group. Sex, diabetes duration and microalbuminuria in type 1 (insulin-dependent) diabetes mellitus. Diabetologia 1987;30:508A.
25 Wiseman MJ, Viberti GC, Mackintosh D, et al: Glycaemia, arterial pressure, and microalbuminuria in type 1 (insulin-dependent) diabetes mellitus. Diabetologia 1984;26:401–405.
26 Mathiesen ER, Oxenboll K, Johansen PA, et al: Incipient nephropathy in type 1 (insulin-dependent) diabetes. Diabetologia 1984;26:406–410.
27 Sampson MJ, Chambers J, Spriggins D, et al: Echocardiographic evidence of relative left ventricular hypertrophy in type 1 (insulin-dependent) diabetic patients with microalbuminuria. Diabetologia 1988;31:539A.
28 Jones SL, Mattock MB, Close CE, et al: Lipid abnormalities in microalbuminuric type 1 (insulin-dependent) diabetes. Diabetologia 1988;31:505A.
29 Viberti GC, Wiseman MJ: The kidney in diabetes: Significance of the early abnormalities. Clin Endocrinol Metab 1986;15:753–782.
30 Mogensen CE, Christensen CK: Predicting diabetic nephropathy in insulin-dependent patients. N Engl J Med 1984;311:89–93.
31 The Kroc Collaborative Study Group: Blood glucose control and the evolution of diabetic retinopathy and albuminuria. N Engl J Med 1984;311:365–372.

32 Feldt-Rasmussen B, Mathiesen E, Deckert T: Effect of two years of strict metabolic control on progression of incipient nephropathy in insulin-dependent diabetics. Lancet 1986;ii:1300–1304.
33 Marre M, Leblanc CH, Suarez L, et al: Converting enzyme inhibition and kidney function in normotensive diabetic patients with persistent microalbuminuria. Br Med J 1987;294:1448–1452.
34 Christensen CK, Mogensen CE: Antihypertensive treatment: Long-term reversal of progression of albuminuria in incipient diabetic nephropathy. A longitudinal study of renal function. J Diab Complic 1987;1:45–52.
35 Cohen D, Dodds R, Viberti GC: Effect of protein restriction in insulin-dependent diabetics at risk of nephropathy. Br Med J 1987;294:795–798.
36 Wiseman MJ, Hunt R, Goodwin A, et al: Dietary composition and renal function in healthy subjects. Nephron 1987;46:37–42.
37 Oakley WG, Pyke DA, Tattersall RB, et al: Long-term diabetes: a clinical study of 92 patients after 40 years. Q J Med 1984;43:145–156.
38 Viberti GC, Keen H, Wiseman MJ: Raised arterial pressure in parents of proteinuric insulin-dependent patients. Br Med J 1987;295:575–577.
39 Mangili R, Bending JJ, Scott G, et al: Increased sodium-lithium countertransport activity in red cells of patients with insulin-dependent diabetes and nephropathy. N Engl J Med 1988;318:146–150.
40 Krolewski AS, Canessa M, Warram JH, et al: Predisposition to hypertension and susceptibility to renal disease in insulin-dependent diabetes mellitus. N Engl J Med 1988;318:140–145.

Prof. G. C. Viberti, Unit of Metabolic Medicine, 4th Floor Hunts House,
Guy's Hospital, GB-London SE1 9RT (UK)

Oldrizzi L, Maschio G, Rugiu C, et al. (eds): The Progressive Nature of Renal Disease: Myths and Facts. Contrib Nephrol. Basel, Karger, 1989, vol 75, pp 127–133

Weighted Least Square Regression Analysis of Factors Contributing to Progression of Chronic Renal Failure[1]

Mackenzie Walser

Department of Pharmacology and Molecular Sciences and Department of Medicine, Johns Hopkins University, Baltimore, Md., USA

Since we first reported anecdotally [1] that nutritional therapy may slow progression of chronic renal failure, there has been growing interest in two possibilities: (1) that a common mechanism causes progression of many types of chronic renal failure, and (2) that this process can be slowed or arrested by diet or drugs.

Recently, we have reported [2] that 5 patients progressing on this diet supplemented with essential amino acids exhibit slowed or arrested progression when changed to ketoacids, suggesting a specific effect of ketoacids on progression.

Previously we have reported that branched-chain ketoacids, especially 2-ketoisocaproate, exert protein-sparing effects [3–5]. One way in which these two different effects of ketoacids might be related is suppression of glucocorticoid production. Glucocorticoids play a role in the regulation of protein turnover [6, 7]. Even though they are often used therapeutically in chronic renal disease, it is conceivable that their beneficial immunological effects at high dosage might obscure a deleterious effect on progression within the physiological range of hormone production, mediated perhaps by an effect on renal protein turnover.

In the present study this hypothesis was tested by measuring progression in patients with renal failure, and relating it to some of the above-mentioned factors postulated to contribute to progression and to glucocorticoid production. The latter was measured as 24-hour urinary excretion rate of 17-hydroxycorticosteroids (17-OHCS) [8].

[1] Supported by a Research Grant (DK-32008) and a Clinical Center Grant (RR-00722) from the National Institutes of Health. This article is adapted from a recent article: Walser M, Ward L: Progression of chronic renal failure is related to glucocorticoid production. Kidney Int 1988;34:859–867, but includes additional data and employs weighted regression analysis.

Materials and Methods

Multiple regression analysis of the factors determining progression rate was performed, based on longitudinal observations during treatment periods lasting an average of 13 months, in 36 patients (23 males and 13 females) with chronic renal failure. Age varied from 23 to 78 years (mean 53 years). Diagnoses were: diabetic nephropathy, 9; glomerulonephritis, 13; interstitial nephritis, 4; polycystic kidney disease, 6; unknown, 4. Patients with IgA nephropathy were excluded because of the variable course of this disorder [9, 10]. Ten patients were treated by mild protein restriction alone. The others were prescribed a diet [2] containing 0.3 g/kg ideal weight of protein and 7–9 mg/kg ideal weight of phosphorus, supplemented with vitamins. However, 24-hour urinary urea N analyses showed that compliance was poor and protein consumption was in fact higher, averaging about 0.56 g/kg. In 18 studies, subjects received a mixture of ketoacids and amino acids, described in detail elsewhere [2], at a dose of 18 g/day. In the remaining 20 studies, patients received a mixture of essential amino acids [2] at a dose of 10 g/day. Ten patients received first amino acids and then ketoacids. All were seen monthly or bimonthly. Blood pressure was measured at each visit in the sitting posture by a single observer, and averaged over the entire study. All but 4 patients received anti-hypertensive drugs, including enalapril in 13 studies. Diuretics were required in all but 6, sodium polystyrene sulfonate in 5, $NaHCO_3$ in 8, and aluminum-containing antacids in 3. All received $CaCO_3$, 2–3 g/day. Twenty-four-hour urine samples were obtained without a preservative, and were kept in a refrigerator during and after collection.

Fasting serum and 24-hour urine chemical values were measured in the Johns Hopkins Hospital Chemistry Laboratory. 17-OHCS excretion was measured in the Pediatric Endocrine Laboratory, using the Silber-Porter method [8]. Glomerular filtration rate (GFR) was measured bimonthly as the urinary clearance of intravenously injected ^{99m}Tc-DTPA (100 μCi). Correction for body weight or surface area was not made. Progression was calculated as the linear regression of GFR on time in months. Pretreatment values were not employed, in order to exclude bias introduced by a possible acute decrease in GFR in response to reduction of protein intake. The average number of bimonthly GFR determinations was 5.8 (minimum 3). Mean starting GFR was 13 ml/min.

Serum and urine chemical values were averaged over the entire period of observation in each subject. An average of 5 measurements of 17-OHCS was obtained in each subject.

The data were analyzed by weighted multiple linear regression, using as independent variables in the primary analysis the quantities listed in table 1, including 'dummy variables', i.e. variables scored as 0 or 1: sex, ketoacid therapy, enalapril therapy and each of the four diagnoses listed above. The 48 studies were considered as independent observations for simplicity, even though 10 patients were studied twice. Weighted multiple linear regression was carried out using a stepwise technique [11]. First, the one-variable model yielding the highest F statistic was computed. Additional variables were added one by one, using a significance level of 0.05 as a criterion for entry. After a variable was added, all variables were reexamined and any were deleted that did not produce an F statistic significant at the 0.05 level. For weights, the reciprocal of the variances of the estimates of progression rate in each study were employed.

Results

Simple Correlation between Progression Rate and 17-OHCS Excretion. When progression rate was examined as a function of all 19 variables, 17-OHCS was the most significant regressor. This linear relationship is

Table 1. Independent variables examined in multiple regression analysis

Continuous variables
17-OHCS excretion, µg/day
Urea N excretion, g/day
Phosphorus excretion, mg/day
Protein excretion, g/day
Serum calcium times phosphorus, mg^2/dl^2
Serum alkaline phospatase, IU/l
Serum uric acid, mg/dl
Serum cholesterol, mg/dl
Serum triglycerides, mg/dl
Mean arterial pressure, mm Hg
Age, years
'Dummy' variables
Sex
Ketoacid therapy
Enalapril therapy
Diabetic nephropathy
Interstitial nephritis
Chronic glomerulonephritis
Polycystic kidney disease

shown in figure 1 as the solid line. Similar linear relationships between progression and 17-OHCS were seen in each of the three treatment subgroups.

Results of Weighted Multiple Regression Analysis. The results are shown in table 2. 17-OHCS excretion accounted for 42% of the variation in progression rate, and was a highly significant regressor ($p < 0.0001$). Proteinuria and phosphaturia were also correlated with progression rate, being greater in those progressing more rapidly, and accounting for 9.8 and 4.9%, respectively, of the variation in progression. Patients with polycystic kidney disease progressed more rapidly, on the average (by 0.28 ml/min/month), than the others ($p = 0.0041$). Suprisingly, higher values for mean arterial pressure were associated with slower rates of progression. However, the level of significance ($p = 0.016$) was in the borderline range for this type of analysis with multiple variables.

Effect of Treatment. An analysis of variance was performed to compare mean values of each parameter in the three treatment groups, (1) protein restriction alone, (2) amino acids, and (3) ketoacids. Although mean values for GFR and progression rate differed, these differences failed

Table 2. Predictors of progression rate in 48 studies in 36 patients, using weighted least squares multiple regression

Variable	b, ml/min/month	Partial r^2	Model r^2	p
17-OHCS	−0.050	0.423	0.423	0.0001
Proteinuria	−0.057	0.098	0.520	0.0041
Polycystic disease	−0.284	0.114	0.634	0.0006
Mean arterial pressure	+0.007	0.047	0.681	0.016
Phosphaturia	−0.0003	0.049	0.730	0.008

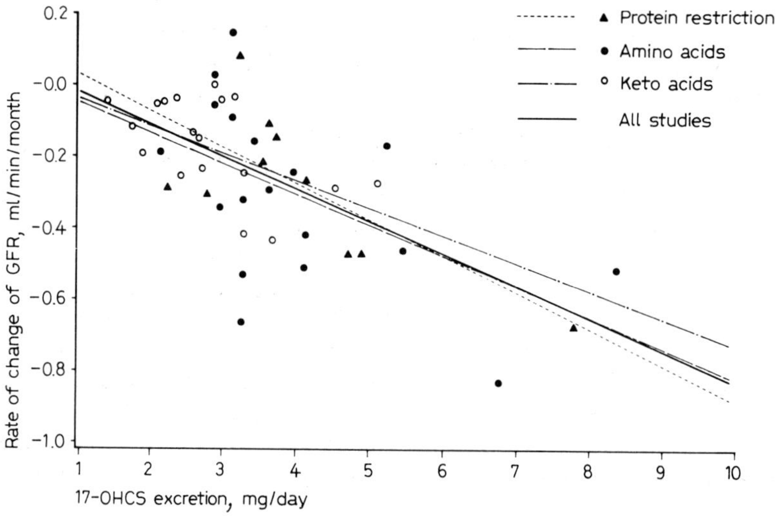

Fig. 1. Rate of change of GFR plotted against 17-OHCS excretion in all studies. The dashed lines represent the linear regression slopes in each of the three treatment groups and the solid line represents the linear regression slope in all studies combined. All of the regressions shown are statistically significant.

to attain statistical difference, as would be expected in this relatively small series. Serum chemical values also did not differ. 17-OHCS differed significantly between the three groups, in the order (1) > (2) > (3). Urinary urea N excretion was the same in the two groups on a severely restricted diet (2 and 3), but was significantly higher in those on mild protein restriction alone (group 1). Mean arterial pressure did not differ between the groups.

Discussion

A relationship between progression of chronic renal failure and endogenous glucocorticoid production has apparently not been reported prior to this work. The correlation found here is highly significant statistically. It does not follow, however, that high levels of glucocorticoids accelerate the progression of chronic renal failure or the converse. Changes in progression and in glucocorticoid production may both be consequences of other unidentified variables.

Wide variation in progression rates among patients with chronic renal failure has long been recognized but never explained. The present relationship provides clues that may prove useful in accounting for this variation. A highly significant correlation between progression rate and 17-OHCS was seen, even in patients not receiving ketoacids. The latter finding appears to exclude the possibility that the correlation seen in all 24 subjects is a spurious consequence of effects of ketoacids to alter glucocorticoid metabolism or renal handling of 17-OHCS.

Several mechanisms by which corticoids might promote progression can be envisaged. For example, glucocorticoids stimulate Na-K-ATPase activity [12], which may play a role in the progression of polycystic kidney disease [13] as well as other types of renal disease. Glucocorticoids inhibit phospholipase A_2 and suppress the production of prostaglandins by renal interstitial cells [14], but in vivo they increase renal prostaglandin production [15], perhaps via lipolytic effects. Eicosanoids cause constriction of glomerular mesangial cells, thereby lowering the glomerular ultrafiltration coefficient [16]. Glucocorticoids at 10 times physiologic dosage increase glomerular capillary pressure in subtotally nephrectomized rats, thereby augmenting glomerular injury, an effect prevented by the administration of angiotensin-converting enzyme inhibitors [17]. Glucocorticoids may increase proteinuria in patients with chronic renal disease [18–20]. However, it should be noted that the 17-OHCS excretion rates observed in the present study are all within (or in a few cases below) the normal range, defined in this laboratory as 2–9 μg/day. Hence steroid effects seen only at pharmacologic dosage may not be relevant to the present relationship. Obviously endogenous glucocorticoids do not damage the normal kidney.

Variations within the normal range of glucocorticoid activity have been shown to have profound effects on protein turnover. Simmons et al. [6] found an increase in proteolysis in human subjects during infusion of sufficient cortisol to increase the plasma level fourfold. Legaspi et al. [7] reported that release of essential amino acids from the human forearm increased fourfold on infusing enough cortisol to raise plasma cortisol less than fourfold. Clark [21] noted that adrenalectomized rats retain more dietary nitrogen than sham-operated controls. How protein turnover and progression might be related is not clear.

Conceivably, the reportedly beneficial effect of protein restriction alone on the progression of chronic renal failure [22] may also be related to lower glucocorticoid production. A high-protein intake has been reported to increase plasma cortisol throughout the day in normal subjects [23] and protein-containing midday meals stimulate cortisol secretion [24]. In normal subjects as well as in the patient studies reported previously, we have confirmed that protein restriction reduces daily 17-OHCS excretion [unpublished data].

Suppression by ketoacids of glucocorticoid production, at least in patients with chronic renal failure, is strongly suggested by these data. Whether such an effect is demonstrable in normal subjects remains to be determined, as well as whether suppression of secretion of adrenocorticotrophic hormone or corticotropin-releasing hormone occurs. Since we have previously found that 2-ketoisocaproate, the analogue of leucine, spares nitrogen in fasting [3, 4] and postoperative man [5], it is likely that this component of the mixture of ketoacids used here is the one responsible for inhibiting glucocorticoid production. If so, slowing of progression might be induced by this compound alone. The present data are not sufficient to establish the component responsible for the effects observed, nor the time course of the effect.

References

1 Walser M: Ketoacids in the treatment of uremia. Clin Nephrol 1975;3:180–187.

2 Walser M, LaFrance ND, Ward L, et al: Progression of renal failure in patients given ketoacids following amino acids. Kidney Int 1987;32:123–126.

3 Sapir DG, Walser M: Nitrogen-sparing induced early in starvation by infusion of branched-chain ketoacids. Metabolism 1977;26:301–308.

4 Mitch WE, Walser M, Sapir DG: Nitrogen sparing induced by leucine compared to that induced by its keto analogue, alpha-ketoisocaproate, in fasting obese man. J Clin Invest 1981;67:553–562.

5 Sapir DG, Stewart PM, Walser M, et al: Effects of alpha-ketoisocaproate and of leucine on nitrogen metabolism in post-operative patients. Lancet 1983;i:1010–1014.

6 Simmons PS, Miles JM, Gerich JE, et al: Increased proteolysis. An effect of increases in plasma cortisol within the physiologic range. J Clin Invest 1984;73:412–420.

7 Legaspi A, Albert JD, Calvano SE, et al: Proteolysis of skeletal muscle in response to acute elevation of plasma cortisol in man. Surg Forum 1985;36:16–17.

8 Silber RH, Porter CC: The determination of 17, 21-dihydroxy-20-ketosteroids in urine and plasma. J Biol Chem 1954;210:923–932.

9 Magil AB, Ballon HS: IgA nephropathy–evaluation of prognostic factors in patients with moderate disease. Nephron 1987;47:246–252.

10 D'Amico G: The commonest glomerulonephritis in the world–IgA nephropathy. J Med 1987;64:709–728.

11 SAS User's Guide: Statistics, ed 5. SAS Institute, 1985, p 764.
12 Ellis D, Tran SD, Avner ED: Glucocorticoid-induced stimulation of Na-K ATPase activity in tubular epithelial cells is mediated by glucocorticoid receptors (GR). Kidney Int 1987;31:165.
13 Avner ED, Sweeney WE, Young MC, et al: Na-K ATPase activity modulates congenital murine polycystic kidney disease in vitro. Clin Res 1987;35:542A.
14 Grunfeld JP, Eloy L, Araujo A, et al: Effects of gluco- and antiglucocorticoids on renal and aortic prostaglandin synthesis. Am J Physiol 1986;251:F810–816.
15 Erman A, Nasjletti A: Enhancement of renal medulla prostaglandin synthetase activity by dexamethasone treatment in the rat. Biochem Biophys Res Commun 1984;121:255–260.
16 Dunn M: The role of arachidonic acid metabolites in renal homeostasis. Non-steroidal anti-inflammatory drugs, renal function and biochemical, histological and clinical effects and drug interactions. Drugs 1987;33(suppl 1):56–66.
17 Garcia DL, Rennke HG, Brenner BM, et al: Chronic glucocorticoid therapy amplifies glomerular injury in rats with renal ablation. J Clin Invest 1987;80:867–874.
18 Heymann W, Grupe WE: Increase in proteinuria due to steroid medication in chronic renal disease. Pediatrics 1969;74:356–363.
19 Dowdle E, Saunders SJ: The acute effect of hydrocortisone sodium succinate on the proteinuria of the nephrotic syndrome. S Afr J Lab Clin Med 1957;3:39–47.
20 Wetzels JFM, Gerlag PGG, Sluiter HE, et al: Prednisone-induced fluctuations of proteinuria in patients with a nephrotic syndrome. Nephron 1986;44:344–350.
21 Clark I: The effect of cortisone on protein synthesis. J Biol Chem 1953;200:69–76.
22 Acchiardo SR, Moore LW, Cockrell S: Does low protein diet halt the progression of renal insufficiency? Clin Nephrol 1986;25:89–94.
23 Sellini M, Fierro A, Marchesi L, et al: Comportamento dei valori dei base e del ritmo circadiano dello ACTH, del cortisolo, della PRL e del GH nel corso di dieta iperproteica. Boll Soc It Biol Sper 1981;57:963–969.
24 Ishizuka B, Quigley ME, Yen SSC: Pituitary hormone release in response to food ingestion: Evidence for neuroendocrine signals from gut to brain. J Clin Endocrinol Metab 1983;57:1111–1116.

Mackenzie Walser, MD, Johns Hopkins University School of Medicine,
Department of Pharmacology and Molecular Sciences, 725 N. Wolfe Street,
Baltimore, MD 21205 (USA)

Oldrizzi L, Maschio G, Rugiu C, et al. (eds): The Progressive Nature of Renal Disease: Myths and Facts. Contrib Nephrol. Basel, Karger, 1989, vol 75, pp 134–140

Protein-Restricted Diet in Early Chronic Renal Failure

Giuseppe Maschio, Lamberto Oldrizzi, Carlo Rugiu
Division of Nephrology, University Hospital, Verona, Italy

In this paper we shall focus on the following points: (1) the results of an early versus a late administration of a protein-restricted diet, and (2) the clinical effects of this diet in patients with chronic renal failure.

Early versus Late Treatment

Both dietary and nondietary intervention have been suggested for preventing progression of chronic renal disease. Dietary measures include restriction of protein, phosphate and salt and supplementation with polyunsaturated fatty acids. Nondietary intervention is based on the administration of antihypertensive agents, dopamine agonists, anticoagulant agents, immunosuppressive drugs and, obviously, insulin in diabetic nephropathy.

In the last 2 years, experimental evidence has been provided that dietary protein and phosphate restriction and selective antihypertensive treatment – applied when renal injury is severe and longstanding – may not be successful in ameliorating the progressive course of chronic renal disease. The extent to which adaptive alterations in glomerular hemodynamics and/or structural changes were already established may have blunted, or averted, the expected results of both dietary and pharmacologic intervention in these studies. Conversely, a therapeutic approach at earlier stages has been proved to exert a more protective role on renal function and structure [1–6].

Extrapolating from experimental studies to therapeutic strategies in human renal disease is usually risky. Some clinical evidence, however, seems to support the critical role of an early therapeutic approach in patients with chronic renal disease and some clinical data were already available before the experimental studies were performed.

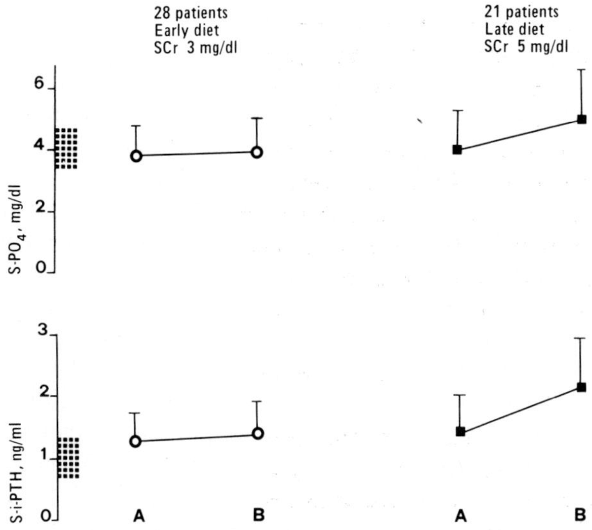

Fig. 1. A = Baseline; B = after 2 years of diet.

We have long been convinced that the degree of functional renal deterioration was critical in modulating the effects of dietary phosphate (and protein) restriction. Our assumption was originally based on the results obtained by this dietary regimen in the control of hyperphosphatemia and in the prevention of secondary hyperparathyroidism. The long-term administration of a low-phosphate, low-protein diet was more effective in patients with a serum creatinine (SCr) level of about 3.0 mg/dl than in those with more advanced renal failure [7, 8] (fig. 1).

Studies along these lines have eventually shown that the effect of phosphate restriction on the renal synthesis of $1{,}25(OH)_2$ vitamin D is strictly dependent on the levels of glomerular filtration rate (GFR) at which it is started, being absent when GFR is below 20 ml/min [9].

Early prevention of hyperphosphatemia may help to avert functional deterioration as well. Increased renal calcium deposition has been shown to occur early in the course of renal disease and could be demonstrated in patients with SCr of less than 1.5 mg/dl who had histologic evidence of renal disease, the major determinant of this early nephrocalcinosis being transient or persistent hyperphosphatemia [10].

On the other hand, several studies from independent laboratories have shown an inverse correlation between the renal hemodynamic compliance and the degree of renal failure, suggesting that when renal injury is severe and longstanding a maximal adaptive response, and hence a relative insensitivity of GFR to dietary protein manipulation, occur in remnant glomeruli [11–13].

In 1979 we reported the results of two groups of patients with chronic renal failure of diverse etiology treated with dietary protein and phosphate restriction. In group 1, SCr concentration rose from a mean level of 3.10 to 6.35 mg/dl over 4 years. In group 2, consisting of 20 patients with earlier renal failure, there was practically no change in SCr over 18 months. In the same group of patients, there was a good correlation between changes in SCr and in GFR (evaluated as renal clearance of iothalamate) over 24 months [8, 14].

Several additional studies have eventually supported the importance of an early dietary approach. Bennet et al. [15], after grouping the patients according to their renal function at the start of low-protein diet, obtained the best results in those with SCr of less than 7.4 mg/dl and suggested that dietary modifications should be introduced early to obtain maximum response.

From a prospective study in 20 patients with early chronic renal failure, Giordano [16] came to the conclusion that the dietary approach is especially useful when initiated at plasma creatinine levels of about 2.0 mg/dl. A plasma creatinine level of 2.8 mg/dl was found to be the crucial point in the progression of renal disease: when this level is reached, the process of nephron loss is accelerated.

Surprisingly, we reached almost the same conclusion in a larger population of patients followed for longer periods of time. At the start of a low-protein diet, SCr and phosphate values were significantly higher in patients who eventually had progression of functional deterioration than in those who had stable renal function. The percentage of patients with no progression of renal failure was maximal when the diet was started at SCr values of about 2.0 mg/dl [17].

With a more sophisticated statistical analysis – using the Cox's proportional hazard model – in 390 patients with chronic renal failure of diverse etiology, starting a dietary protein restriction at SCr levels of 3.0 mg/dl was associated with a relative risk of renal death (SCr = 10 mg/dl) four times higher than that observed when dietary treatment was started at an SCr level of 2.0 mg/dl. Accordingly, the actuarial survival probability at 84 months was 86.4% when SCr on entry was lower than 2.0 mg/dl; it decreased to 60.9% when SCr ranged between 2.0 and 3.0 mg/dl; and it fell to 41.6% at SCr levels exceeding 3.0 mg/dl [18].

Finally, in a randomized clinical trial, Locatelli [19] observed a much better cumulative proportional survival in patients treated with a low-protein diet at early stages of renal failure than in those with SCr exceeding 5.0 mg/dl. Thus, the available clinical experience suggests that the earlier the dietary approach the better is the probability of survival in terms of renal function.

Clinical Effects with Protein-Restricted Diet

After some earlier reports showing positive effects of low-protein diets – with or without amino acid supplementation – on the course of renal failure [20–23], in the last 6 years several clinical studies on the effects of low-protein diets, unsupplemented with essential amino acids, in patients with chronic renal failure, have been published. They include a one-group design with nonequivalent comparison, self-controlled studies, randomized crossover studies, and randomized clinical trials [24–36].

Virtually all these reports have concluded that protein restriction slowed the progression of renal disease, and almost all of them have been criticized for being retrospective, uncontrolled, or methodologically inadequate. Major criticism has been expressed on the techniques to measure progression. They include rate of change of SCr, creatinine clearance, survival curves and isotope GFR (or insulin clearance).

According to Walser [37], reliable estimates of progression can be made only be sequential measurements of isotope GFR, or insulin clearance, and the traditional use of creatinine measurements for diagnosing and following patients with chronic renal failure may no longer be supportable.

From a practical viewpoint, however, SCr – sequentially evaluated some months after the institution of a low-protein diet, when a new metabolic setting has been achieved – is still a good index of renal function. On these conditions, the day-to-day coefficient of variation is small (6.5%) and, therefore, acceptable [38]. Iothalamate clearance was frequently measured in our patients in steady-state conditions and did not show substantial difference as compared to SCr determinations. On the other hand, it should be remembered that SCr is still the universally used biochemical parameter for deciding when patients are to be started on regular dialysis treatment.

Between 1974 and 1988, we have studied 390 patients with chronic renal failure of diverse etiology. Their SCr at the start was 2.26 ± 1.10 mg/dl and the average follow-up is now 54 ± 28 months. The clinical results were expressed using the following criteria: 222 patients (57%) had stable renal function (no change in SCr or its increase of less than 0.02 mg/dl/month); 42 patients (11%) had slow deterioration of renal function (increase in SCr exceeding 0.02 but lower than 0.04 mg/dl/month); and 126 patients (32%) had fast deterioration of renal function; their increase in SCr exceeding 0.04 mg/dl/month. Thus, progression of renal failure was virtually halted in more than two thirds of the patients for almost 5 years.

As expected [17], the nature of underlying renal disease, the severity of hypertension, the degree of proteinuria, the presence of the nephrotic syndrome and the late administration of the diet were the most important factors responsible for the progressive deterioration in the minority of patients. All patients had excellent compliance with the diet, as evaluated with the current techniques, and the large majority of them also had a good nutritional state.

Conclusions

These results explain why we did not randomize our patients on purpose. We are aware of the validity of well-conducted randomized clinical trials, but we were prevented from doing so by the perhaps too many variables (age, sex, underlying renal disease, magnitude of proteinuria, presence of the nephrotic syndrome, duration and severity of hypertension, degree of functional deterioration on entry, rate of progression of renal failure before randomization) that should be considered when the assignment of patients between treated or untreatead groups is to be made, and by the feeling that strict randomization was not acceptable in our patients.

We still feel that the scientific ideal – which incorporates both randomization and blinding – is less important than routine treatment if this treatment is able to keep constant SCr levels for many years in the large majority of patients, is well accepted by patients, and is not harmful to them.

References

1 Nath KA: Dietary protein restriction in established renal injury in the rat. J. Clin Invest 1986;78:1199–1205.
2 Lumlertgul D: Phosphate depletion arrests progression of chronic renal failure independent of protein intake. Kidney Int. 1986;29:658–666.
3 Meyer TW: Reversing glomerular hypertension stabilizes established glomerular injury. Kidney Int 1987;31:752–759.
4 Beukers JB: Converting enzyme inhibition and progressive glomerulosclerosis in the rat. Kidney Int 1987;32:794–800.
5 Hirschel-Scholtz S: Protection from progressive renal failure and hyperparathyroidism bone remodeling by WR-2721. Kidney Int 1988;33:934–941.
6 Motomura K: Importance of early initiation of dietary protein restriction for the prevention of experimental progressive renal disease. Nephron 1988;49:144–149.

7 Fiaschi E: Low-protein diets and bone disease in chronic renal failure. Kidney Int 1978;13(Suppl 8):S79–S82.
8 Maschio G: Early dietary phosphorus restriction and calcium supplementation in the prevention of renal osteodystrophy. Kidney Int 1980;23:1546–1554.
9 Tessitore N: Relationship between serum vitamin D metabolites and dietary intake of phosphate in patients with early renal failure. Miner Electrolyte 1987;13:38–44.
10 Gimenez LF: Relation between renal calcium content and renal impairment in 246 human renal biopsies. Kidney Int 1987;31:93–99.
11 Bosch JP: Short-term protein loading in assessment of patients with renal disease. Am J Med 1984;77:873–879.
12 Rodriguez-Iturbe B: Response to acute protein load in kidney donors and in apparently normal postacute glomerulonephritis patients: evidence for glomerular hyperfiltration. Lancet 1985;i:461–464.
13 Ter Wee PM: Tesing renal reserve filtration capacity with amino acid solution. Nephron 1985;41:193–199.
14 Maschio G: Effects of dietary protein and phosphorus restriction on the progression of early renal failure. Kidney Int 1982;22:371–376.
15 Bennett, B: Low protein diets in uraemia. Br Med J 1983;287:1344–1345.
16 Giordano C: Early dietary protein restriction protects the failing kidney. Kidney Int 1985;17 (Suppl 17):66–70.
17 Maschio G: Factors affecting progression of renal in patients on long-term dietary protein restriction. Kidney Int 1987;32(Suppl 22): 49–52.
18 Oldrizzi L: The Verona experience on the effect of diet on progression of renal failure. 5th Int. Congr on Nutrition and Metabolism in Renal Disease. Strasbourg, September 1988.
19 Locatelli F: Controlled study of protein restricted diet in chronic renal failute. 2nd Verona Seminar on Nephrology. September 1988.
20 Kluthe R: Clinical aspects of amino acid metabolism in renal disease. Clin Nutr 1985;4 (spec suppl):3.
21 Walser M: Urea metabolism in chronic renal failure. J Clin Invest 1974;53:1385–1392.
22 Walser M: Ketoacids in the treatment of uremia. Clin Nephrol 1975;3:180–186.
23 Walser M: The effect of nutritional therapy on the course of chronic renal failure. Clin Nephrol 1979;11:66–70.
24 Maschio G: Effects of dietary protein and phosphorus restriction on the progression of early renal failure. Kidney Int 1982;22:371–376.
25 Barsotti G: Restricted phosphorus and nitrogen intake to slow the progression of chronic renal failure: a controlled trial. Kidney Int 1983;24(Suppl 16):S278–S284.
26 Oldrizzi L: Progression of renal failure in patients with renal disease of diverse etiology on protein restricted diet. Kidney Int 1985;27:553–557.
27 Acchiardo SR: Does low protein diet halt the progression of renal insufficiency? Clin Nephrol 1986;25:289–294.
28 Evanoff GV: The effect of dietary protein restriction on the progression of diabetic nephropathy. Arch Intern Med 1987;147:492–495.
29 El Nahas AM: Selective effect of low-protein diets in chronic renal disease. Br Med J 1984;289:1337–1341.
30 Schaap GH: The effect of a high protein intake on renal function of patients with chronic renal insufficiency. Nephron 1987;47:1–6.
31 Oldrizzi L: Effects of two different protein diets on progression of early chronic renal failure: a self-controlled study. Proc 20th ASN Meet, Dec 1987.

32 Viberti GC: Low protein diets and progression of diabetic kidney disease. Nephrol Dial Transpl 1988;3:334–339.
33 Rosenberg ME: Effect of protein intake on glomerular function in human renal disease. Kidney Int 1986;29:A325.
34 Rosman JB: Prospective randomized trial of early dietary protein restriction in chronic renal failure. Lancet 1984;ii:1291–1296.
35 Zeller KR: The effect of dietary protein modification on renal function in diabetic nephropathy. Kidney Int 1987;31:225–230.
36 Williams AJ: Effect of varying quantity and quality of dietary protein intake in experimental renal disease in rats. Nephron 1987;46:83–90.
37 Walser M: Progression of renal failure. Proc 10th Int Congr of Nephrology. London, Saunders, 1988, pp 1155–1181.
38 Fraser CG: Short-term biological variations of plasma analytes in renal disease. Clin Chem 1983;29:508–515.

Giuseppe Maschio, MD, Division of Nephrology, Ospedale Civile Maggiore, I–37126 Verona (Italy)

Oldrizzi L, Maschio G, Rugiu C, et al. (eds): The Progressive Nature of Renal Disease: Myths and Facts. Contrib Nephrol. Basel, Karger, 1989, vol 75, pp 141–146

Controlled Study of Protein-Restricted Diet in Chronic Renal Failure

Francesco Locatelli[1]

Divisione di Nefrologia e Dialisi, Ospedale di Lecco, Italia

The prevention of renal disease progression is still a challenge to medical science as well as a growing social and economic problem. The ever-improving knowledge of the physiopathological mechanisms involved in renal diseases in animal models has shown some effective ways of slowing down or preventing the progression of chronic renal failure. Low-protein (LP) diets have been prescribed for many years for the symptomatic relief of uraemic symptoms [1]. More recently it has been claimed that a LP diet may also slow down or halt the progression of renal failure [2, 3].

There is striking evidence that this is true in experimental renal failure produced in rats by subtotal nephrectomy or glomerulonephritis [4, 5]. Nevertheless, there are differences between strains of rats as well as between species (rats, rabbits, dogs) in terms of their susceptibility to progressive renal failure following extensive nephrectomy.

Does restriction of dietary protein slow down the progression of renal disease in man? Many reports show that this seems to be the case. However the results obtained in experimental studies must be checked in man by means of controlled clinical trials. Until now there has been a dearth of good controlled data and only one prospective randomized trial [3].

In 1983, we decided to plan a multicentre, controlled, randomized, prospective and adequately sized trial on the effects of LP diet on the progression of chronic renal failure. The trial started in April 1984 and the recruiting period lasted until May 1985.

The aim was to evaluate in a large controlled randomized trial the effects of a LP diet (0.6 g/kg/die) in comparison with a controlled-protein diet (CP, 1 g/kg/die) on patients with chronic renal failure. Both diets also foresaw a phosphorus restriction.

[1] On behalf of the Northern Italy Cooperative Study Group for the Conservative Treatment of Chronic Renal Failure.

Protocol Presentation[2]

Study Design. This was an open, multicentre, between-patient, prospective trial, with centrally randomized allocation of the two diets. The patients were stratified into three groups according to plasma creatinine values (PlCr): group A, ≥ 1.5 (1.35 in women) and < 2.5 mg/dl; group B, ≥ 2.5 and < 5.0 mg/dl; group C, ≥ 5.0 and < 7.0 mg/dl. The duration of the study was set at 24 months on LP or CP diet after a 3-month period of preliminary observation.

Inclusion Criteria. Patients of both sexes, aged from 18 to 65 years with values of PlCr ranging from 1.5 (1.35 in women) to 7.0 mg/dl and GFR < 60 ml/min, calculated according to the Cockroft formula, were considered eligible for the study. Written informed consent was also required.

Exclusion Criteria. Patients with nephrotic syndrome (serum albumin < 2.5 g/dl; proteinuria > 3 g/l), diabetes, recent myocardial infarction, acute renal failure, acute obstruction and infection of urinary tract, systemic diseases and previous gastro-intestinal resection surgery were excluded. Patients showing doubling of PlCr values within the 3-month preliminary observation period were also excluded.

Dietetic Prescriptions. The LP diet foresaw a daily protein intake of 0.6 g/kg (0.5 animal), with caloric supply of 35 kcal/kg and a phosphorus intake of 8 mg/kg while the CP diet foresaw a daily protein intake of 1.0 g/kg (0.6 animal), with caloric supply of 30 kcal/kg and a phosphorus intake of 13 mg/kg. Dietary intake was calculated on the basis of ideal body weight according to Broca's formula.

Concomitant Treatments. Calcium supplements and phosphate binders (preferably calcium carbonate) were given in order to maintain normal values of calcaemia and phosphataemia. Vitamin D was not allowed. The maintenance of blood pressure values below 150/90 mm Hg, using antihypertensive drugs, was recommended avoiding ACE inhibitors.

Assessments. Clinical and laboratory assessments were performed 3 months before admission to the study (preliminary period) and every 3 months thereafter throughout the study. An additional clinical assessment was performed one month after the assignment of the diet. A survey of the routine dietetic inquiries was performed by a skilled dietician every 6 months on one third of the patients, randomly chosen.

Evaluation Criteria. The slope of reciprocal creatinine plots and the behaviour of the PlCr and creatinine clearance values were originally considered as evaluation criteria for the progression of renal failure. But, later on, following the many criticisms of the use of the

[2] *Steering Committee:* F. Locatelli (Chairman), D. Alberti, M.G. Gentile, G. Graziani, G. Buccianti, G. Cairo, P. Cosci. *Participating Centres:* Lecco (F. Locatelli), Milano-San Carlo (G. D'Amico), Milano-Croff (C. Ponticelli), Milano-Granelli (G. Buccianti), Monza (B. Redaelli), Busto Arsizio (A. Giangrande), Varese (L. Gastaldi), Bergamo (G. Mecca), Milano-S. Paolo (D. Brancaccio), Desio (A. Confalonieri), Pavia (A. Salvadeo), Lodi (M. Surian), Vimercate (A. Sessa), Melegnano (C. Grassi), Pinerolo (A. Ramello), Cremona (F. Pecchini), Mantova (C. Baroni), Cinisello (F. Vallino), Novara (G. Verzetti), Brescia-Umberto I (A. Castellani), Modena (E. Lusvarghi). *Ethical Committee:* G. Maschio, G. Tognoni, P.C. Zucchelli. *Statistical Analysis:* B.M. Francucci (Ciba-Geigy Medical Dept.-Italy).

Table 1. Primary renal disease of patients admitted into the study

	Group			Total (%)
	A	B	C	
Glomerulonephritis	61	59	12	132 (29.0)
Nephroangiosclerosis	40	27	5	72 (15.8)
Interstitial nephropathy	81	59	16	156 (34.2)
Polycystic kidney	26	30	18	74 (16.2)
Others (Alport's syndrome malformations)	8	12	2	22 (4.8)
	216	187	53	456 (100)

Group A: plasma creatinine (PlCr) ⩾1.5 (1.35 in women) and <2.5 mg/dl; group B: PlCr ⩾2.5 and <5 mg/dl; group C: PlCr ⩾5 and <7 mg/dl.

Table 2. Distribution of patients according to plasma creatinine (PlCr) values and assigned diet

Group	LP diet	CP diet	Total
A	107	109	216
B	99	88	187
C	24	29	53
	230	226	456

Group A: PlCr ⩾1.5 (1.35 in women) and <2.5 mg/dl; group B: PlCr ⩾2.5 and <5 mg/dl; group C: PlCr ⩾5 and <7 mg/dl.

reciprocal creatinine slope, renal survival curves were taken into account in order to evaluate the progression of renal failure. The following end-points were considered as criteria of renal non-survival: doubling of initial PlCr values or need for dialysis. The results of the dietary inquiries and urinary urea and phosphorus values were used to check patient compliance.

Statistical Analysis. The homogeneity of patient distribution between centres and between diets was checked by means of the χ^2 test for non-parametric data and 1-way ANOVA for parametric data.

For the efficacy analysis the following tests were used: log rank test (Breslow and Mantel-Cox survival curves); analysis of variance according to a split-plot design; linear regression and correlation; non-parametric tests for qualitative data.

Patients. 456 patients, 247 men and 209 women, were admitted into the study. Their mean age was 48.5 years (range 18–65). Distribution according to primary renal disease is shown in table 1. Table 2 shows the distribution of patients according to PlCr values and assigned diet.

Preliminary Results

Three hundred and eleven patients (68.2%) concluded the follow-up. Seventy-six (16.7%) dropped out of the study (38 on the LP diet and 38 on the CP diet) because of lack of cooperation (58), the onset of concomitant diseases (4), intolerance to LP foods (6), death (5) or other causes (3). To date only the results referring to end-points has been considered: for the other parameters, quality control is still under way. Twenty-seven patients (5.9%) on the LP diet and 42 patients (9.2%) on the CP diet reached an end-point.

As far as the total study population is concerned, cumulative proportional survival, taking end-points as criteria of renal non-survival, is better in patients on the LP diet; although the difference is not significant, it is very near to it ($p = 0.0596$ Breslow, 0.0592 Mantel-Cox). Stratifying according to PlCr values, the difference is again nearly but not significant in group A ($p = 0.0549$ Breslow, 0.0546 Mantel-Cox), but it is very significant in group B ($p = 0.0249$ Breslow, 0.0238 Mantel-Cox). No difference at all was found between the LP and the CP diets in group C.

Discussion

If we examine from the methodological point of view the data published in the literature on the efficacy of protein restriction in slowing down the progression of chronic renal failure, we must say that, unfortunately and for many reasons, the controls used are very often methodologically inadequate. Such controls are actually affected by many systematic errors which frequently invalidate the results.

In 1982, Maschio et al. [2] reported the effects of protein and phosphorus restriction on the progression of early chronic renal failure. In that study, 2 groups of patients with basal creatinine values of 2.18 and 4.2 mg/dl, respectively, underwent protein restriction. They showed a better slope of serum creatinine than a group of patients with free protein intake whose basal serum creatinine was 2.28 mg/dl. The untreated control group was set up retrospectively, using patients from other centres: the follow-up period was also shorter. This makes evaluation of the results difficult, since the groups were selected and followed up in a heterogeneous way.

Similar comments may be made about a successive study from the same authors [6], in which three groups of patients were put on a protein restricted diet, followed prospectively and compared with a group of retrospectively selected patients on a free diet. Nevertheless, due to the size of the study and the consistency of the results, these reports strongly support the hypothesis that hypoproteic diet slows down the progression of renal disease.

In 1984, El Nahas et al. [7] studied the effects of protein restriction (6 months) in patients stratified according to underlying nephropathy: interstitial nephritis (9 patients), glomerulonephritis (12 patients), nephrosclerosis (9 patients) and polycystic kidney (4 patients). The authors concluded that a LP diet was effective in the first group, scarcely effective in the second one and totally ineffective in the last two. Unfortunately, due to the small number of patients, the risk of both type I and type II errors is very high. In fact, patients with a more or less favourable natural clinical course may have been included by chance in each group, and this fact, rather than the diet itself, may have affected the results. The paper by Rosman et al. [3] is the only prospective randomized study to date, in which an adequate number of patients was randomly allocated to protein restriction or free diet and all the patients groups were followed up in the same way. Results showed that the LP diet significantly slowed down the progression of renal failure, in comparison with the control group. However there was no mention of patient compliance, and subsequent papers by the same group [8] have not confirmed these results. In 1986, a paper by El Nahas and Coles [9] appeared in which some criticism was expressed about studies published on the effect of protein restriction. The paper ends by suggesting eight 'recommendations for future studies'. Our study, planned in 1983 and started in 1984 fulfilled all these recommendations, except for renal function monitoring by isotopic clearances. However, in agreement with Giovannetti [10], we think that long periods of follow-up and repeated measurements of creatinine clearances give an adequate assessment of renal function and satisfactorily indicate the rate of decline and possible improvement.

Conclusions

The high social costs of end-stage uraemia require the most effective possible secondary prevention.

To date, controlled randomized studies are the most reliable way of evaluating the effectiveness or ineffectiveness of new therapeutical approaches. With the exception of Rosman et al. [3], none of the studies on protein restriction efficacy published so far have used adequate controls. The preliminary results of our randomized controlled study seems to offer some support to the hypothesis that protein restriction is efficacious in slowing down the progression of renal failure in patients with plasma creatinine values below 5 mg/dl. However, evaluation of the final results and of patient compliance, as well as of the role of other important factors such as proteinuria, blood pressure, calcium-phosphorus product and underlying nephropathy is still under way.

References

1 Giovannetti S, Maggiore Q: A low nitrogen diet with protein of high biological value for severe chronic uremia. Lancet 1964;i:1000–1004.
2 Maschio G, Oldrizzi L, Tessitore N, et al: Effects of dietary protein and phosphorus restriction on the progression of early renal failure. Kidney Int 1982;22:371–376.
3 Rosman JB, ter Wee PM, Meijer S, et al: Prospective randomized trial of early dietary protein restriction in chronic renal failure. Lancet 1984;ii:1291–1296.
4 Ibels LS, Alfrey AC, Haut L, et al: Preservation of function in experimental renal disease by dietary phosphate restriction. N Engl J Med 1978;298:122–126.
5 Hostetter TH, Meyer TW, Rennke HG, et al: Chronic effects of dietary protein in the rat with intact and reduced renal mass. Kidney Int 1986;30:509–517.
6 Oldrizzi L, Rugiu C, Valvo E, et al: Progression of renal failure in patients with renal disease of diverse etiology on protein-restricted diet. Kidney Int 1985;27:553–557.
7 El Nahas AM, Masters-Thomas A, Brady SA, et al: Selective effect of low protein diets in chronic renal disease. Br Med J 1984;289:1337–1341.
8 Rosman JB, Donker AJM: Dietary protein restriction in chronic renal failure: an update. Abstracts 5th Int Congr on Nutrition and Metabolism in Renal Disease. Strasburg 1988, p. 148.
9 El Nahas AM, Coles GA: Dietary treatment of chronic renal failure: ten unanswered questions. Lancet 1986:i:597–600.
10 Giovannetti S: Answers to ten questions on the dietary treatment of chronic renal failure. Lancet 1986;ii:1140–1142.

Francesco Locatelli, MD, Division of Nephrology and Dialysis,
Hospital of Lecco, I–22053 Lecco (Italy)

Oldrizzi L, Maschio G, Rugiu C, et al. (eds): The Progressive Nature of Renal Disease: Myths and Facts. Contrib Nephrol. Basel, Karger, 1989, vol 75, pp 147–154

Supplemented Diet for Severe Chronic Renal Failure: Some Controversial Points

Sergio Giovannetti

Clinica Medica 1, Università di Pisa, Italia

The low-protein, low-phosphorus pure vegetarian diet supplemented with essential amino acids and keto-analogues (supplemented diet) [1] is being introduced in the clinical practice for the management of severe chronic renal failure, and there is a general agreement on its efficacy in preventing and reversing the manifestations of chronic uremia. The still debated questions are: (1) Which is the correct method to assess the rate of progression of renal failure? (2) Does dietary therapy affect the rate of progression? (3) Does dietary treatment cause protein malnutrition? These three points will be examined.

The Measurement of the Residual Renal Function to Evaluate the Rate of Progression of Renal Failure

The discussion on this point refers mostly to the question whether creatinine (Cr) may be used in some way to measure renal function without obtaining misleading informations.

Confusion is often made between serum Cr (sCr) and the reciprocal of sCr (1/sCr), on one side, and Cr clearance (CrCl) on the other. There is a great difference between the former two and the latter, but this is often forgotten.

Both sCr and 1/sCr are largely dependent on the amount of Cr that is produced and, for an equal impairment of renal function, the values of sCr and of 1/sCr are quite different if the production of Cr is different. On low-protein diets and, particularly, on a pure vegetarian diet (not containing Cr nor creatine), the production of Cr is very low, the values of sCr are also low and those of 1/sCr are high.

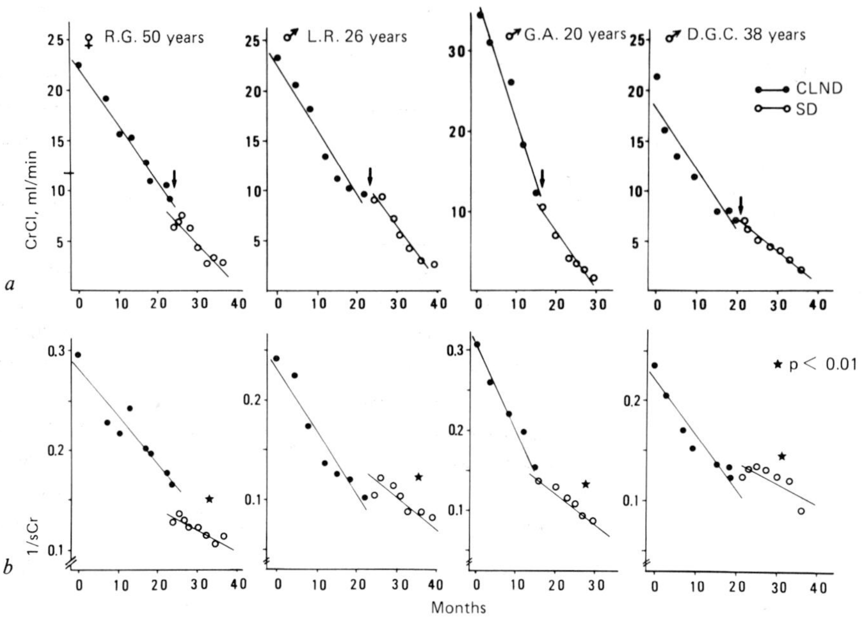

Fig. 1. CrCl rates *(a)* and reciprocal of sCr values *(b)* plotted against time during a period of conventional low-protein diet (black points) and during a period of supplemented diet (circles). Asterisks = existence of a significant difference; arrows = beginning of supplemented diet. The 4 patients were suffering from reflux nephropathy.

The problems with CrCl are completely different. The changes in the production of Cr affect equally both its renal output and its serum concentration and the U.V/P ratio does not change for this.

The difference in the meaning of CrCl and of 1/sCr is shown in figure 1. The slope of the regression lines of the rates of CrCl is not significantly different during the supplemented diet period and during the previous period of conventional low-protein diet, clearly indicating that in these 4 patients (suffering for reflux nephropathy) no change occurred in the rate of progression following the supplemented diet. On the contrary, the regression lines of 1/sCr are significantly different giving misleading information due to the low production of Cr that lower the only denominator of the 1/sCr ratio.

CrCl is higher than the glomerular filtration rate (GFR) and this has been known for several decades [2]; and it is also known that this is due to an active tubular secretion of Cr that increases as the sCr levels increase,

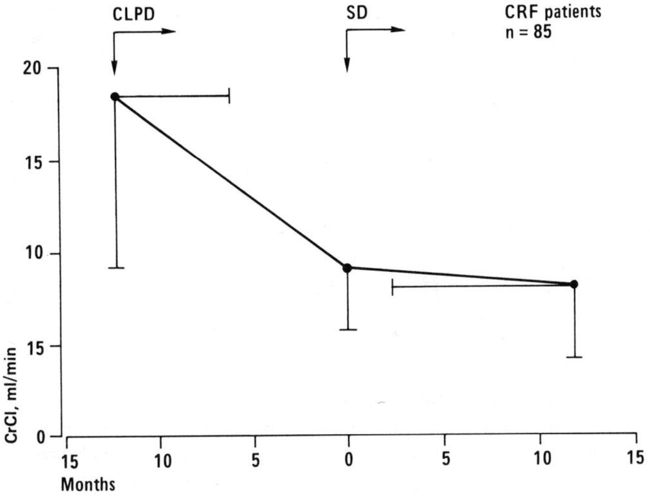

Fig. 2. CrCl rates plotted against time during a period of conventional low-protein diet (CLPD) and during a period of supplemented diet. Eighty-five unselected chronic renal failure patients are reported here.

following venous infusion [3] or following a fall of GFR [4, 5]. The consequences are that a mild renal impairment is not detectable with CrCl and that the changes of GFR are blunted if CrCl is used to measure it. To summarize: CrCl is less sensitive than the measurement of GFR with inulin or with the isotopes.

The information given by CrCl is then not misleading and appears adequate for the purpose of assessing the changes of renal function occurring in the course of many months and even some years of treatment with the supplemented diet.

Effects of the Supplemented Diet on the Rate of Progression of Chronic Renal Failure

The rate of deterioration of residual renal function was assessed with the measurement of CrCl in 81 severe chronic renal patients. All the observed chronic renal diseases and also the noncomplying patients were included in this evaluation: the nonresponders (reflux nephropathy, glomerulonephritis of recent onset) were examined together with the diabetic nephropathy patients who had a very good response [6]. This ac-

Table 1. The clinical state of the studied patients

	Age years	Sex		Body weight, kg	Arterial pressure mean mm Hg
		M	F		
Complying (n = 49)	48.7 ± 12	34	15	60.02 ± 11	118 ± 3.6
Noncomplying (n = 32)	49.6 ± 10	22	10	68.41 ± 9	119 ± 4.4

Table 2. Possible mechanisms of protection of residual renal function

Factors causing progression of chronic renal failure	Nature and frequency	Effects of supplemented diet
1 Glomerular hypertension and hyperfiltration	Virtually constant and very important	Decrease
2 Nephrocalcinosis	Important but occasional	Decrease of the Ca.P product
3 Renal oxalosis	Important but occasional	Decrease of serum oxalate
4 Acidosis with elevated ammonia in kidney tissue	Hypothesis to be demonstrated	Correction
5 Increased traffic of macromolecules in mesangial cells	Hypothesis to be demonstrated	Decrease

counts for the large dispersion of the data but, in spite of this, a flattening of the regression line was observed during the supplemented diet period, as previously reported [1], indicating a slowing of the rate of progression (fig. 2).

In this type of evaluation each patient is the control of himself and it is assumed that the rate of decline is linear with time. To avoid this assumption a second type of evaluation was made on the same data. The 32 noncomplying patients were regarded as controls and the 49 complying patients were regarded as the study patients. The rate of decline of the residual renal function was significantly lower in the complying patients

Duration of treatment months	Initial CrCl ml/min	Rate of deterioration ml/min/month	Daily urinary urea output, g
22.08 ± 13	8.7 ± 2.4	−0.136 ± 0.129	3.23 ± 0.7
13.18 ± 6	8.8 ± 2.9	0.495 ± 0.272	7.71 ± 1.3

than in the controls (noncomplying) (fig. 3). This way to select controls is not orthodox but, considering that the other various parameters (including the incidence of the various renal diseases) were quite similar (table 1), the only variable being diet, the results appear quite convincing.

In conclusion, the rate of deterioration of the residual renal function is often significantly lower in chronic renal failure patients following the supplemented diet than in those who do not adhere to the prescriptions. The possible mechanism(s) through which such effect(s) may be exerted are probably nonspecific for single renal diseases and some of them are indicated in table 2.

The Protein Nutritional Status and Supplemented Diet

Protein malnutrition is a consequence of long-lasting severe chronic renal failure both in the untreated and in the dialyzed patients. Metabolic acidosis [7, 8], hormonal and metabolic derangements and low caloric intake are the main catabolic factors causing malnutrition.

Though these causes are well known, protein malnutrition is usually attibuted to the low-protein intake and the treatment is generally based on the increase of the protein supply. The consequences are a stimulus of the protein anabolism that is, however, counterbalanced by an increase of the catabolic factors. This creates a vicious circle and, consequently, a progressive deterioration of the nutritional state. The rational basis for the prevention and the treatment of protein malnutrition is the removal of the catabolic factors with dialysis therapy or with correct dietary therapy.

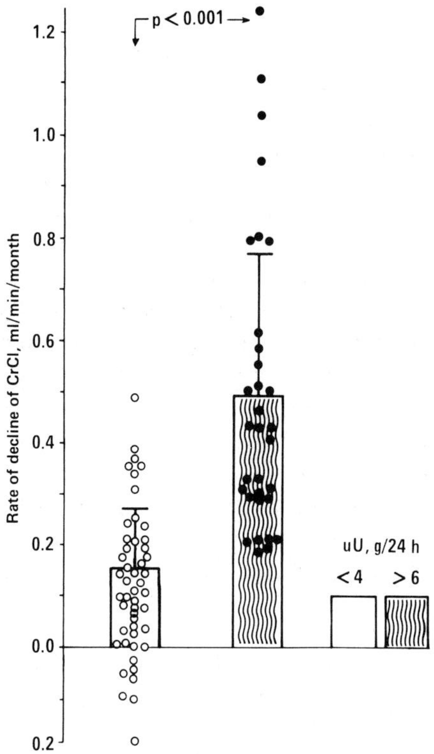

Fig. 3. The rate of decline of CrCl (ml/min/month) in 49 chronic renal failure patients complying to the supplemented diet (circles), and in 49 noncomplying patients (black points), uU = urinary urea. See also table 1.

The supplemented diet completely prevents metabolic acidosis [our unpublished observations], prevents and reverses secondary hyperparathyroidism [9, 10] (fig. 4), male hypogonadism [our unpublished observations] and corrects carbohydrate intolerance [our unpublished observations. (fig. 5)]. These effects of the supplemented diet account for the lack of manifestations of protein malnutrition even after several years. Both the anthropometric measurements (fig. 6) and the rapid turnover serum proteins were found, indeed, to be normal even after 7 years of supplemented diet therapy.

In conclusion, chronic renal failure itself often causes protein malnutrition and the supplemented diet, if correctly planned and carried out, is a valuable measure of prevention.

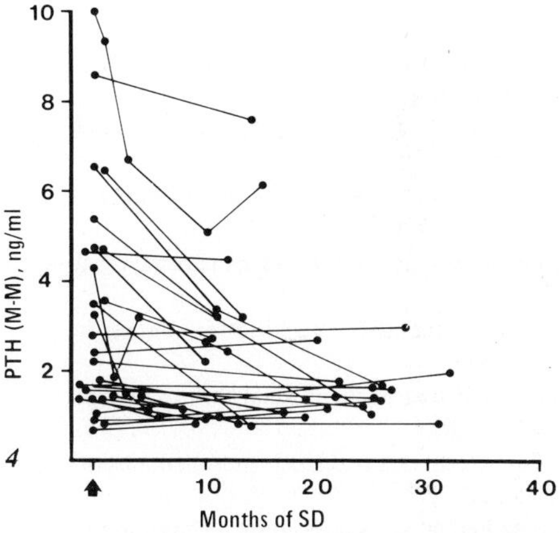

4

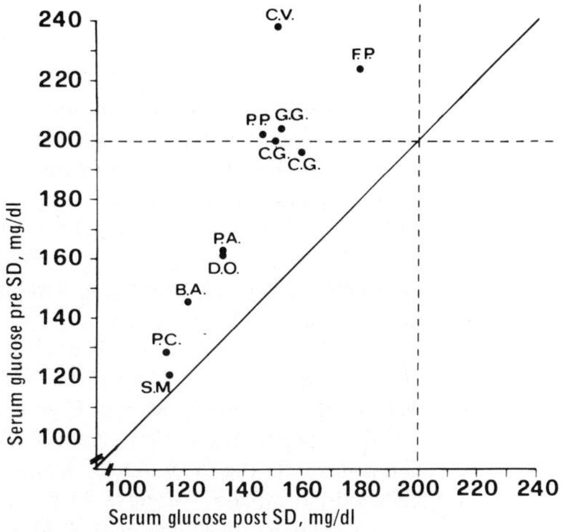

5

Fig. 4. The changes in the serum concentration of parathyroid hormone (middle molecular segment) in 27 chronic renal failure patients following the supplemented diet.

Fig. 5. The maximum serum glucose levels in 11 chronic renal failure patients before and after 3–4 weeks since the beginning of supplemented diet. Oral tolerance test.

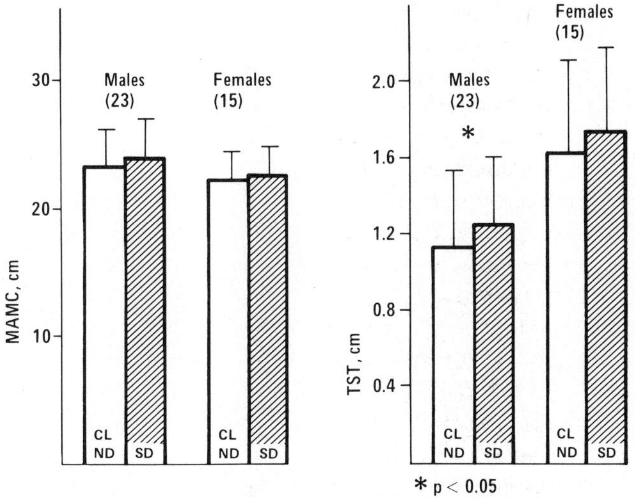

Fig. 6. The behavior of the middle arm muscle circumference (MAMC) and of the triceps skin-fold thickness (TST) in 38 chronic renal failure patients. Mean ± SD.

References

1 Barsotti G, Guiducci A, Ciardella F, et al: Effects on renal function of a low-nitrogen diet supplemented with essential amino acids and ketoanalogues and of hemodialysis and free protein supply in patients with chronic renal failure. Nephron 1981;27:113–117.
2 Smith HW: The Kidney. Structure and Function in Health and Disease. Oxford University Press, New York, 1951, pp 182–194.
3 Miller BF, Winkler AW: The renal excretion of endogenous creatinine in man. Comparison with exogenous creatinine and insulin. J Clin Invest 1938;17:31–39.
4 Giovannetti S, Cioni l, Balestri PL: Evaluation of kidney function in severe chronic renal failure. Urol Dig 1966;5:15–20.
5 Shemesh O, Golbetz H, Kriss JP, et al: Limitation of creatinine as a filtration marker in glomerulopatic patients. Kidney Int 1985;28:830–838.
6 Barsotti G, Ciardella F, Morelli E, et al: Nutritional treatment of renal failure in type 1 diabetic nephropathy. Clin Nephrol 1988;29:280–287.
7 Giovannetti S, Bigalli A, Della Santa M: Gli effetti della acidosi sperimentale sul metabolismo proteico. Minerva Med 1957;48:38–42.
8 Hara Y, May RC, Kell RA, et al: Acidosis, not azotemia, stimulates branch chain amino acids catabolism in uremic rats. Kidney Int 1987;32:808–814.
9 Barsotti G, Morelli E, Guiducci A, et al: Reversal of hyperparathyroidism in severe uremics following a very low-protein and low-phosphorus diet. Nephron 1982;30:310–313.
10 Lindenau K, Kokot F, Fröhling PT: Suppression of parathyroid hormone by therapy with a mixture of ketoanalogues-aminoacids in hemodialysis patients. Nephron 1986;43:84–86.

Sergio Giovannetti, MD, la Clinica Medica Generale e Terapia,
Università di Pisa, Ospedale Santa Chiara, I–56100 Pisa (Italy)

Oldrizzi L, Maschio G, Rugiu C, et al. (eds): The Progressive Nature of Renal Disease: Myths and Facts. Contrib Nephrol. Basel, Karger, 1989, vol 75, pp 155–166

Antihypertensive Therapy and Progression of Renal Failure

Vito M. Campese, Chaplin Liu

Division of Nephrology, Department of Medicine, University of Southern California, Los Angeles, Calif., USA

It is well known that hypertension can cause renal injury both in humans and in animals with congenital or experimentally induced hypertension [1]. Moreover, hypertension frequently develops in patients with renal disease and it may accelerate the progression of renal damage.

Recently, it has been speculated that the variable rate of renal injury caused by the hypertension in different models may largely depend on the functional adaptation of the preglomerular resistance [1].

Thus, the choice of antihypertensive agents should not only be based on their hypotensive efficacy but also on the capacity to favorably affect glomerular hemodynamics.

The purpose of this review is to first analyse the specific relationship between hypertension and intrarenal hemodynamic adaptation in human subjects and in several models of experimental hypertension; the second purpose is to review the current knowledge on the effects of several antihypertensive agents on intrarenal hemodynamics and on the progression of renal diseases.

Functional and Anatomical Renal Abnormalities in Essential Hypertension

Humans

The frequency of clinically significant renal insufficiency in patients with essential hypertension in the absence of an accelerated phase is debated [2–6].

In a postmortem analysis of 420 untreated cases, Bell and Clawson [2] noted a prevalence of renal failure of 8.6%.

Perera [3] evaluated 500 untreated patients with essential hypertension and observed that 18% developed renal insufficiency, and 10% of them died of uremia. Among these patients, 7% had developed malignant hypertension. Several other studies have reported rates of renal failure in patients with essential hypertension ranging from 4 to 20% [4, 5]. Kincaid-Smith [6], on the other hand, found no impairment of renal function above that expected from aging in a group of 131 consecutive cases of benign essential hypertension studied postmortem.

It is common knowledge that black patients with hypertension have an extraordinarily higher relative risk (4–5 times) of developing strokes or end-stage renal disease (ESRD) than white hypertensive patients [7, 8].

Rostand et al. [9] observed that hypertension was the cause of renal failure in 16% of patients with ESRD in a rural county in Alabama. Hypertension was the cause of renal failure more commonly in blacks (30%) than in whites (11%). The average incidence of ESRD was 4.2 times greater in blacks than in whites.

This phenomenon could be in part attributed to a greater propensity of black patients to remain untreated or to have poorly controlled hypertension. An alternative explanation, however, could be that for any given level of blood pressure elevation, the renal or cerebral circulation may be subjected to more severe vascular injuries in blacks than in whites.

Black hypertensive patients have more severe nephrosclerosis than white patients, involving primarily the arcuate renal arteries; they also display less renal blood flow than white hypertensive patients even when age and severity of hypertension are taken into account [10]. Intrarenal arterial disease in blacks with malignant hypertension is also quite different than in whites. Blacks show no evidence of fibrinoid necrosis, the classic lesion of malignant hypertension.

This concept is of extreme importance particularly in light of recent controversies on whether patients with mild hypertension should be treated immediately with antihypertensive agents or whether drug treatment should be withheld for 6–12 months [11, 12]. These questions have been raised since several large Cooperative Trials on the management of mild hypertension have raised the suspicion that pharmacologic therapy may not necessarily have an impact on cardiovascular morbidity and mortality in patients with mild hypertension [13]. These concepts, however, may not necessarily be applicable to hypertensive blacks. The Hypertension Detection and Follow-up Program (HDFP) which comprised 40% black patients showed that 80% of the decreased mortality was due to improved survival among black hypertensive patients [14]. This suggests that untreated mild hypertension could have a worse prognosis in blacks than in white patients and it should, therefore, be treated more aggressively.

Animal Species

It appears that renal function deteriorates faster as a consequence of hypertension in some strains of rats with congenital hypertension than in others.

Wistar-Okamoto spontaneously hypertensive rats (SHR) and Dahl's salt-sensitive rats are two inbred strains genetically predisposed to develop hypertension. The hypertension in SHR develops spontaneously whereas in Dahl's predisposed rats hypertension develops only when the animals are fed a diet with high sodium content. At approximately 1 year of age SHR have proteinuria, glomerular sclerosis and reduced glomerular filtration rate (GFR) [14]. These lesions, however, affect predominantly the juxtaglomerular nephrons, whereas the superficial nephrons are relatively spared [14]. On the contrary, the kidneys of Dahl's salt-sensitive rats are more susceptible to glomerulosclerosis [15].

Mechanisms of Glomerular Injury in Human and Experimental Hypertension

Recent evidence indicates that the variable rate of progression of glomerular injury in these various models of hypertension in rats may be in large part related to adaptation of preglomerular vascular resistance.

There is a common belief that hypertension exerts its damaging effects on the kidneys through vasoconstriction and/or arteriolar vascular sclerosis which in turn would lead to glomerular ischemia and sclerosis. Recently, however, this concept has been challenged primarily on the basis of studies which have allowed one to measure intrarenal hemodynamics in a number of experimental models of hypertension. These studies have demonstrated that a failure of arteriolar constriction of the afferent glomerular arterioles rather than progressive narrowing may be responsible for direct transmission of hypertension to the glomeruli leading to progressive injury [1].

In hypertensive SHR the preglomerular arteriolar resistance is increased, thus maintaining normal intraglomerular pressure despite a rise in systemic blood pressure. In these rats the kidneys appear to be relatively protected and have lesser progression of glomerular sclerosis.

On the other hand, Dahl's salt-sensitive rats have reduced preglomerular vascular resistance while glomerular blood flow, glomerular capillary pressure and single-nephron glomerular filtration rate (SNGFR) are increased [1]. These hemodynamic changes in early stages in life in Dahl's rats maintain a normal GFR despite a congenital reduced number of nephrons but, later on, they may cause progressive glomerular injury and sclerosis.

The alterations of intrarenal hemodynamics in human essential hypertension are less well understood. Most patients display an increase in renal vascular resistance.

Hollenberg et al. [16] have demonstrated variable and significant abnormality of renal blood flow in patients with essential hypertension depending on their age. Bianchi et al. [17] have shown an increase in renal blood flow in human subjects during the prehypertensive state. Messerli et al. [18] have shown increased, normal or diminished renal blood flow in patients with borderline hypertension which was related to the cardiac output.

In older patients with advanced glomerulosclerosis, renal blood flow decreases and it is not significantly affected by intrarenal administration of vasodilators [19]. This suggests that the renal vascular abnormalities in advanced nephrosclerosis are largely fixed and related to organic changes.

The GFR is usually normal or slightly decreased in patients with essential hypertension, giving an increased filtration fraction. With the persistance of uncontrolled hypertension, renal blood flow may continue to decrease largely as a consequence of sclerotic changes in afferent arterioles. To maintain GFR, efferent arteriolar tone and intraglomerular pressure may increase further. This may create a vicious circle causing the progressive demise of glomeruli.

Goldrin et al. [20] observed in 60 hypertensive patients with established essential hypertension a decrease in renal blood flow which was related to the severity of hypertension. They also suggested that the increase in resistance in the efferent arterioles was greater than in the afferent arterioles and that this maintained GFR. This type of adaptation would also imply an increase in intraglomerular pressure.

Lowenstein et al. [21] based on indirect estimation of renal interstitial pressure concluded that human subjects with essential hypertension display a rise in intraglomerular pressure despite increased afferent arteriolar resistance.

On the other hand, Gomez [22] calculated that the predominant change in the renal circulation of patients with essential hypertension is an increase in afferent arteriolar resistances.

No data are available on whether intrarenal hemodynamics vary during the course of the disease in patients with essential hypertension. It is theoretically possible that different adaptation of intraglomerular hemodynamics may account for the variable rate of progression of renal failure in patients of different races, in the same way as variable adaptations occur in different strains of spontaneously hypertensive rats.

It is also possible that the progressive loss of nephrons may concur to changing intraglomerular hemodynamics during the course of the disease.

Hypertension and Progression of Glomerular Diseases

Hypertension develops frequently in patients with glomerulonephritis and it may play a major role in the progression of glomerulosclerosis even when the initiating immunologic events have subsided. The degree of renal vascular sclerosis observed in patients with chronic glomerulonephritis are usually more severe than those observed in patients with essential hypertension having comparable levels of blood pressure [1]. On the basis of experimental evidence it has been suggested that the accelerated course of vascular and glomerular damage in patients with hypertension and renal parenchimal disease might be due to enhanced transmission of hypertension to glomeruli having dilated afferent arterioles as an adaptive mechanism in the setting of reduced nephron mass.

Baldwin and Neugarten [1] have studied the influence of two-kidney one-clip hypertension on the course of mild nonprogressive nephrotoxic serum nephritis. They observed vascular and glomerular sclerosis which were not recorded in animals with nephritis in the absence of hypertension or with hypertension without nephritis. Glomerular capillary pressure and transcapillary hydraulic pressure difference were increased both in kidneys with nephrotoxic nephritis as well as in kidneys with hypertension. However, when nephritis and hypertension were associated, glomerular capillary pressure and transcapillary hydraulic pressure increased even further. These alterations may explain the increased vascular and glomerulosclerosis in models in whom hypertension and glomerulonephritis are combined.

The rate of progression of renal failure induced by immune mediated glomerulonephritis in animals with preexisting spontaneous hypertension also varies depending on whether or not systemic hypertension is transmitted to the glomerular capillaries. Immune-mediated glomerulonephritis induced in SHR leads only to mild glomerulosclerosis; this may be due to the fact that preglomerular vascular resistance increases and intraglomerular pressure does not rise. On the contrary, Dahl's salt-sensitive rats or SHR after uninephrectomy develop severe glomerular damage for similar levels of systemic blood pressure as SHR with intact kidneys [23]. This may be a consequence of reduced preglomerular vascular resistance in this strain of hypertensive rats leading to a further rise of intraglomerular pressure [23].

A model of hypertension associated with renal failure which has been widely studied is that produced by surgical reduction of renal mass. Surgical ablation of renal mass leads to significant changes in intrarenal hemodynamics which may contribute to the progressive sclerosis of the remnant glomeruli. These hemodynamic changes include a decrease in both afferent and efferent arteriolar vascular resistance, increased plasma flow rate and GFR and increased glomerular capillary pressure.

Treatment of Hypertension and Progression of Renal Disease

Mild to Moderate Hypertension

Since the impact of mild to moderate hypertension on the genesis of progressive glomerulosclerosis is debatable, the effects of antihypertensive treatment on renal function are difficult to assess.

Among 380 patients with mild to moderate hypertension evaluated in the Veterans Administration Cooperative Study, renal insufficiency developed in 3 patients treated with placebo and in none of the patients treated with medications [24].

Magee et al. [25] also observed that treatment had no significant effect on renal function in patients with mild to moderate hypertension.

Parving et al. [26] have described an increase in urinary albumin excretion in patients with essential hypertension and conversely a reduction in albumin excretion after blood pressure control.

Hypertension Associated with Renal Diseases

While it is well established that hypertension may accelerate the progression of renal disease, only few controlled studies have been performed to determine the impact of effective antihypertensive therapy on the course of these diseases. Two retrospective studies [27, 28] showed that control of hypertension effectively reduced the rate of renal functional deterioration in patients with glomerulonephritis. More recently, Bauer and Gaddy [29] have shown that converting-enzyme inhibitors (CEI) or calcium channel blockers [30] were able to control blood pressure and (in the short-term) to stabilize renal function in patients with renal insufficiency. Some preliminary studies have also suggested that therapy with CEI may be more effective than conventional treatment in reducing the progression of renal disease [31].

Antihypertensive Agents and Renal Function

To study the effect of antihypertensive agents on the kidneys is extremely important for two reasons. First, since the kidney exerts a pivotal role in the genesis and/or maintenance of any form of hypertension independent of its etiology [32], the ability of an antihypertensive agent to sustain a decrease in blood pressure depends in large part on its effects on renal function. Second, the specific effects of an antihypertensive agent on intrarenal hemodynamics may influence the progression of renal insufficiency. The choice of specific antihypertensive agents based on their influence on intrarenal hemodynamics may be of great importance in hypertensive patients with reduced renal mass or with renal parenchimal disease, where the deranged intrarenal hemodynamics appear to play a more significant role in the progression of glomerulosclerosis and of renal insufficiency.

Nonspecific Vasodilators

This class includes hydralazine, diazoxide, sodium nitroprusside and minoxidil. These agents cause renal vasodilatation and no significant effects on GFR [33]. Despite the favorable effect on renal vascular resistance, these agents cause significant sodium retention which may offset the favorable effect on peripheral vascular resistance and mitigate the hypotensive action. The mechanisms responsible for sodium retention have not yet been defined but the decrease in blood pressure, the activation of the renin-angiotensin system and direct renal tubular effects may all play a role [34].

The impact of these agents given alone on the progression of renal injury in human subjects or in animals with experimental hypertension is unknown.

The effects of prolonged minoxidil therapy on glomerular filtration rate in hypertensive patients are variable and may depend on the etiology of hypertension, on the preexisting degree of renal function and on the presence or absence of malignant hypertension. A review of the cases reported in the literature [35–37] showed that minoxidil given for more than 5 months stabilized renal function in the majority (95%) of patients with essential hypertension and normal renal function. However, renal function deteriorated in 23% of patients with essential hypertension and baseline creatinine greater than 1.5 mg/dl and in 52% of patients with renal parenchymal diseases and baseline serum creatinine levels greater than 1.5 mg/dl [38].

Since minoxidil is usually used in combination with other antihypertensive agents, it is unclear whether the beneficial effect on renal function observed during treatment with minoxidil is due to other agents. Moreover, it is unclear if the beneficial effect of minoxidil are only and exclusively related to better control of arterial pressure or to other mechanisms.

Converting Enzyme Inhibitors [39]

The antihypertensive activity of these agents is primarily dependent upon inhibition of the conversion of angiotensin I to angiotensin II.

Since angiotensin II plays a role in the pathogenesis of hypertension in a large number of patients with impaired renal function, it is not surprising that CEI are very effective antihypertensive agents in these patients. Angiotensin II also exerts an important direct influence on renal perfusion pressure, glomerular dynamics, tubular function and, possibly, sympathetic neurotransmission to the kidneys.

CEI increase renal blood flow without any significant change in GFR. Since angiotensin II constricts predominantly the efferent arterioles, CEI result in a decrease in filtration fraction and in glomerular capillary pressure.

This action of CEI may be particularly useful in the management of hypertension accompanying reduction of renal mass.

In the renal ablation model CEI cause a striking reduction in proteinuria and glomerular sclerosis in the remaining tissue compared to rats with a similar degree of renal ablation but receiving placebo [40]. The improvement in the progression of renal lesions was not solely due to reduction of systemic hypertension; in fact when normotension was achieved with a triple therapy (reserpine, hydralazine and hydrochlorothiazide) proteinuria and progression of renal failure were not arrested in this experimental model [41].

CEI but not triple therapy caused significant efferent arteriolar dilatation and a decrease in glomerular capillary pressure [41]. CEI are more efficacious in preventing renal injury in some other hypertensive models, such as in rats with glomerulonephritis [42] or diabetes [43]. On the other hand, triple therapy normalized systemic blood pressure and glomerular capillary pressure and prevented renal injury in uninephrectomized SHR [44]. Captopril was unable to slow the progression of renal disease in adriamycin-induced nephrotic syndrome in rats [45].

Based on the experimental evidence it can be speculated that the aim of antihypertensive therapy in patients with hypertension and reduced renal mass should be not only to reduce systemic pressure, but also to decrease glomerular pressure.

Several clinical studies support this concept. Heeg et al. [46] have compared the effect of lisinopril with that of conventional antihypertensive treatment in patients with renal disease of different origin. Lisinopril reduced proteinuria by 61% whereas conventional therapy had no effect on protein excretion. A significant positive correlation was present between the decrease in urinary protein excretion and the fall in filtration fraction, suggesting a fall in glomerular capillary pressure.

Reams and Bauer [47] have shown that the short-term administration of enalapril to patients with GFR between 9 and 48 ml/min caused an increase in renal blood flow, no change in GFR and a decrease in filtration fraction. On the other hand, prolonged administration of enalapril in patients with GFR less or equal to 80 ml/min caused a 50% increase in GFR at one year and a 33% increase at 3 years. Effective renal plasma flow increased by 33% at 1 and 3 years. Filtration fraction and urinary protein excretion were unchanged [48].

Calcium Channel Antagonists

Acute administration of calcium channel antagonists caused an increase in renal blood flow, in GFR and in urinary sodium, calcium and phosphorus excretion [49, 50]. Long-term therapy with these agents does not normally cause changes in these parameters. The effects of these agents on intrarenal hemodynamics are debated. On the one hand, some have shown a primary vasodilatory action at the level of the afferent arterioles [51]. On the other hand, Frolich [52] has found that the calcium channel antagonist diltiazem produced an increase in renal blood flow and a stable GFR without hyperfiltration. The authors suggested that diltiazem may reverse the abnormalities in efferent arteriole tone in genetically mediated hypertension.

Ichikawa et al. [53] have shown that verapamil normalizes glomerular capillary pressure after it had been raised by infusion of angiotensin II. Besides these potentially beneficial glomerular hemodynamic actions, these agents should at least theoretically reduce the progression of glomerular injury also by virtue of other actions discovered in other cell systems. Recent studies on cell culture have shown that calcium antagonists interfere with the activation of platelets [54] and decrease the release of platelet-activating factor from leukocytes [55]. Heinle and Reich [56] have recently shown that verapamil prevents growth-promoting effects of serum on cultured vascular smooth muscle cells [56]. Therefore calcium channel antagonists may exert a beneficial effect on the progression of renal disease by reducing glomerular hypertension and by interfering with the inflammatory response in the glomerulus.

References

1 Baldwin DS, Neugarten J: Blood pressure control and progression of renal insufficiency; in Mitch WE, Brenner BM (eds): The Progressive Nature of Renal Disease, London, Churchill-Livingstone, 1986, pp 81–110.
2 Bell ET, Clawson BJ: Primary (essential) hypertension: A study of four hundred and twenty cases. Arch Pathol 1928;5:939.
3 Perera G: Hypertensive vascular disease: Description and natural history. J Chron Dis 1955;1:33.
4 Papper J, Vaamonde CA: Nephrosclerosis; in Strauss MB, Welt LB (eds): Diseases of the Kidney, ed 2. Boston, Little, Brown, 1971, vol 2, pp 735–768.
5 Hunter A, Rogers DH: Mortality study of impaired lives, No. 2. Trans Acta Soc AM 1923;24:378.
6 Kincaid-Smith P: The kidney: A clinico-pathological study. Oxford, Blackwell, 1975.
7 Easterling RE: Racial factors in the incidence of causation of end-stage renal disease (ESRD). Trans Am Soc Artif Intern Organs 1977;23:28–32.

8 Dustan HP, Curtis JJ, Luke RG, et al: Systemic hypertension and the kidney in black patients. Am J Cardiol 1987;60:731–771.
9 Rostand SG, Kirk KA, Rutsky EA, et al: Racial differences in the incidence of treatment for end-stage renal disease. N Engl J Med 1982;306:1276–1279.
10 Levy SB, Talner LB, Coel MN, et al: Renal vasculature in essential hypertension: Racial differences. Ann Intern Med 1978;88:12–16.
11 Fries ED: Should mild hypertension be treated? N Engl J Med 1982;307:306–309.
12 Narins RG: Mild hypertension: A therapeutic dilemma. Kidney Int 1984;26:881–894.
13 MacMahon SW, Cutler JA, Furberg CD, et al: The effects of drug treatment for hypertension on morbidity and mortality from cardiovascular disease: A review of randomized controlled trials. Prog Cardiovasc Dis 1986;29(suppl 1):99–108.
14 Hypertension Detection and Follow-up Program Cooperative Group: Five years findings of the Hypertension Detection and Follow-up Program. I. Reduction in mortality of persons with high blood pressure, including mild hypertension. JAMA 1979;242:2562–2571.
15 Azar S, Johnson MA, Hertel B, et al: Single-nephron pressures, flows and resistances in hypertensive kidneys with nephrosclerosis. Kidney Int 1977;12:28–40.
16 Hollenberg NK, Borucki LJ, Adams DF: The renal vasculature in early essential hypertension: Evidence for a pathogenetic role. Medicine 1978;57:167–178.
17 Bianchi G, Cusi D, Guidi E: Renal hemodynamics in human subjects and in animals with genetic hypertension during the prehypertensive stage. Am J Nephrol 1983;3:73–79.
18 Messerli FH, Garavaglia GE, Schmieder RE, et al: Disparate cardiovascular findings in men and women with essential hypertension. Ann Intern Med 1987;107:158–161.
19 Hollenberg NK, Adams DF, Solomon H, et al: Renal vascular tone in essential and secondary hypertension. Hemodynamic and angiographic responses to vasodilators. Medicine 1975;54:29–44.
20 Goldring W, Chasis H, Ranges HA, et al: Effective renal blood flow in subjects with essential hypertension. J Clin Invest 1941;20:637–653.
21 Lowenstein J, Beranbaum ER, Chasis H, et al: Intrarenal pressure and exaggerated natriuresis in essential hypertension. Clin Sci 1970;38:359.
22 Gomez DM: Evaluation of renal resistances with special references to changes in essential hypertension. J Clin Invest 1951;30:1143–1155.
23 Raij L, Azar S, Keane WF: Role of hypertension in progressive glomerular immune injury. Hypertension 1985;7:398–404.
24 Veterans Administration Cooperative Study Group on antihypertensive agents: Effects of treatment on morbidity in hypertension. II. Results in patients with diastolic blood pressure averaging 90 through 114 mm Hg. JAMA 1970;213:1143.
25 MaGee JH, Under AM, Richardson DW: Changes in renal function associated with drug or placebo therapy of human hypertension. Am J Med 1964;36:795–804.
26 Parving HH, Mogensen CE, Jensen HA, et al: Increased urinary albumin-excretion rate in benign essential hypertension. Lancet 1974;i:1190–1192.
27 Fujise Y, Miyahara M: Comparison of the prognosis of hypertension associated with chronic glomerulonephritis with that of essential hypertension. Jpn Circ J 1975;39:793.
28 Kajitwara N: Therapy and prognosis of hypertension in chronic nephritis. Jpn Circ J 1975;39:779.
29 Bauer JH, Gaddy P: Effects of enalapril alone, and in combination with hydrochlorothiazide, on renin-angiotensin aldosterone, renal function, salt water excretion, and body fluid composition. Am J Kidney Dis 1988;4:222–232.
30 Sunderrajar S, Reams G, Bauer JH: Renal vascular changes are reversible with diltiazem. J Hypertens 1986;4(suppl 5):S448–S450.

31 Rulope LM, Miranda B, Miranda B, et al: Control of hypertension with a converting enzyme inhibitor slows progression of renal insufficiency in human chronic renal failure. Kidney Int 1987;31:215.
32 Guyton AC, Coleman TG, Cowley AW Jr, et al: Arterial pressure regulation overriding dominance of the kidneys in long-term regulation and in hypertension. Am J Med 1972;52:584–594.
33 Hollenberg, NK: Vasodilators, antihypertensive therapy, and the kidney. Circulation 1987;75(suppl V):V39–V42.
34 Zins GR: Alterations in renal function during vasodilator therapy; in Wesson LB, Fanelli BN (eds): Recent Advances in Renal Physiology and Pharmacology. Baltimore, University Park Press, 1974, pp 165–186.
35 Campese VM, Stein D, DeQuattro V: Treatment of severe hypertension with minoxidil: Advantages and limitations. Clin Pharmacol 1979;19:231–241.
36 Andersson O, Sivertsson R: Renal function and vascular resistance during long-term minoxidil treatment of severe hypertension. J Cardiovasc Pharmacol 1980;2(suppl 2):123–130.
37 Camel GH, Carmody SE, Perry HM: Use of minoxidil in the azotemic patient. J Cardiovasc Pharmacol 1980;2(suppl 2):173–180.
38 Campese VM: Minoxidil: A review of its pharmacological properties and therapeutic use. Drugs 1981;22:257–278.
39 Zimmerman BG, Wong PC: Alterations in renal function produced by angiotensin converting enzyme inhibitors; in Horovitz ZP (ed): Angiotensin Converting Enzyme Inhibitors. Mechanisms of Action and Clinical Implications. Baltimore, Urban & Schwarzenberg, 1981, pp 239–253.
40 Meyer TW, Anderson S, Rennke HG, et al: Reversing glomerular hypertension stabilized established glomerular injury. Kidney Int 1987;31:752–759.
41 Anderson S, Rennke HG, Brenner BM: Therapeutic advantage of converting enzyme inhibitors in arresting progressive renal disease associated with systemic hypertension in the rat. J Clin Invest 1986;77:1993–2000.
42 Raij L, Chiou X, Owens R, et al: Therapeutic implications of hypertension-induced glomerular injury. Comparison of enalapril and a combination of hydralazine, reserpine, and hydrochlorothiazide in an experimental model. Am J Med 1985;79(suppl 3C):37–41.
43 Zatz R, Dunn BR, Meyer TW, et al: Prevention of diabetic glomerulopathy by pharmacological amelioration of glomerular capillary hypertension. J Clin Invest 1986;77:1925–1930.
44 Dworkin L, Grosser M, Feiner H, et al: Both converting enzyme inhibitors and vasodilators reduce glomerular capillary pressure and injury in uninephrectomized spontaneously hypertensive rats (abstract). Kidney Int 1987;31:383A.
45 Hall RL, Wilke WL, Pettman MJ: The progression of adriamycin-induced nephrotic syndrome in rats and the effect of captopril. Toxicol Appl Pharmacol 1986;82:164–174.
46 Heeg JE, DeJong PE, Van Der Hem GK, et al: Reduction of proteinuria by angiotensin converting enzyme inhibition. Kidney Int 1987;32:78–83.
47 Reams GP, Bauer JH: Effect of enalapril in subjects with hypertension associated with moderate to severe renal dysfunction. Arch Intern Med 1986;146:2145–2148.
48 Bauer JH, Reams GP, Lal SM: Renal protective effect of strict blood pressure control with enalapril therapy. Arch Intern Med 1987;147:1397–1400.
49 Baba T, Boku A, Ishizaki T, et al: Renal effects of nicardipine in patients with mild-to-moderate essential hypertension. Am Heart J 1986;111:552–557.
50 Bauer JH, Sunderrajan S, Reams G: Effects of calcium entry blockers on renin angiotensin-aldosterone system, renal function and hemodynamics, salt and water excretion and body fluid composition. Am J Cardiol 1985;56:62H–67H.

51 Romero JC, Raij L, Grander JP, et al: Multiple effects of calcium entry blockers on renal function in hypertension. Hypertension 1987;10:140–151.
52 Frolich ED: Efferent glomerular arteriolar constriction: a possible intrarenal hemodynamic defect in hypertension. Am J Med Sci 1988;295:409–413.
53 Ichikawa I, Miele JF, Brenner BM: Reversal of renal cortical actions of angiotensin II by verapamil and manganese. Kidney Int 1979;16:136–147.
54 Mehta JL: Influence of calcium channel blockers on platelet function and arachidonic acid metabolism. Am J Cardiol 1985;56:1588–1648.
55 Benviste J: Effect of the Ca-antagonist nefedipine on the release of platelet activating factor (PAF-Acetether), slow-reacting substance and beta-glucuronidase from human neutrophils. Eur J Pharmacol 1983;89:19–26.
56 Heinle H, Reich A: Inhibition by verapamil of the medium-change induced stimulation of cultured vascular smooth muscle cells. Arzneimittel forsch 1985;35:1811-1812.

Vito M. Campese, MD, University of Southern California,
Division of Nephrology, 2025 Zonal Avenue, GNH-4250,
Los Angeles, CA 90033 (USA)

Oldrizzi L, Maschio G, Rugiu C, et al. (eds): The Progressive Nature of Renal Disease: Myths and Facts. Contrib Nephrol. Basel, Karger, 1989, vol 75, pp 167–176

Control of Hypertension and Progression of Chronic Renal Failure

A. Albertazzi, P. Cappelli, B. Di Paolo
Institute of Nephrology, G. D'Annunzio University, Chieti, Italy

The rate of progression to end-stage renal failure of the primary renal diseases is due to several factors in addition to the pathogenetic mechanism intrinsic to the nephropathies themselves. Even when the initial disease is no longer active, increased pressure and flow acting on remnant glomerular capillaries may be responsible for progressive glomerular sclerosis [1].

The natural history, common to all chronic nephropathies, may be affected by other factors accelerating the course of chronic renal failure. These include poorly controlled hypertension, infection or obstruction of the urinary tract, nephrotoxic substances, hyperuricemia and a high Ca × P product [2, 3]. Hypertension is believed to contribute as a main factor in the progression of both experimental and clinical renal diseases [4].

Hypertensive Glomerular Damage in Chronic Renal Failure

The mechanism of progressive nephron loss due to hypertension superimposed on existing glomerular damage has been assumed to relate to glomerular and tubular ischemia secondary to narrowing of small vessels. However recent studies indicate that a hemodynamic, rather than ischemic, mechanism is responsible for accelerating the progression of chronic renal failure due to hypertension [4]. An ischemic mechanism certainly present in accelerated hypertension, because of a significant recent increase over previous hypertensive levels, can originate an obstructive artheriopathy at least in part due to acute injury with spasm and edema of the vessel wall. As this injury resolves, following a good control of blood pressure by drugs, renal function will usually improve [5, 6].

This trend is exemplified in figure 1 where it is schematically represented the clinical course of blood pressure, serum creatinine and fundus oculi in a young female patient affected with chronic glomerulonephritis.

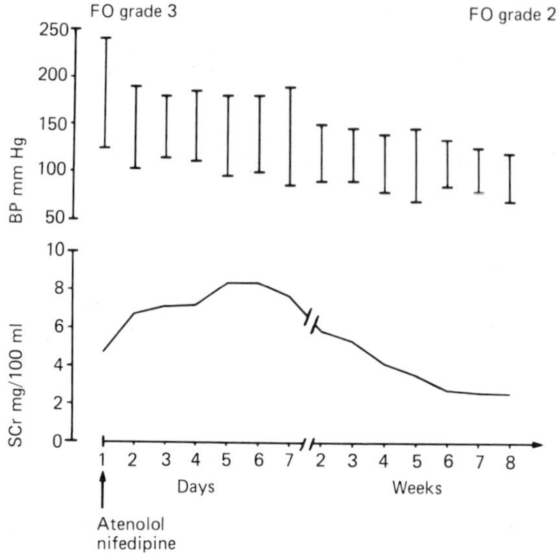

Fig. 1. Clinical course of blood pressure, plasma creatinine and fundus oculi in a young female patient affected with chronic glomerulonephritis and superimposed accelerated hypertension.

She was admitted to the hospital with uncontrolled blood pressure (240/130 mm Hg). She started a hypotensive therapy with β-blockers and calcium-channel antagonists that decreased the blood pressure levels but meanwhile induced a deterioration of renal insufficiency. A few weeks later she got an improvement in renal failure and serum creatinine stabilized at levels lower than before. Concerning the hemodynamic mechanism, numerous experimental data [4, 7] confirm that failure of afferent arteriolar resistance to increase in hyperfiltering nephrons may be responsible for hypertensive damage through increased transmission of elevated systemic pressure to glomerular capillary bed in chronic nephropathies. A low-protein diet may reduce intraglomerular pressure and flow, thus slowing down the progression of morphologic changes [8, 9]. On the other hand, experimental studies on animals and clinical observations in humans [4, 10, 11] confirm that the development of renal damage can be delayed by good control of arterial pressure. The best results seem to be achieved by the use of converting enzyme inhibitors (CEI) which, unlike the conventional antihypertensive treatment, could exert a protective effect on the kidney due to a reduction in glomerular hypertension [12, 13].

Role of Systemic and Glomerular Hypertension in the Progression of Chronic Renal Failure

The effects of low-protein diet and antihypertensive therapy on glomerular damage caused by arterial hypertension in patients with chronic renal failure were evaluated.

Patients and Methods

Two separate studies were conducted. In the first one we carried out a retrospective examination of 37 patients (23 males, 14 females, age 18–66 years) affected with chronic renal failure due to chronic glomerulonephritis. During the follow-up period, which varied from 18 to 70 months, they all presented a linear decline with time of 1/serum creatinine. The patients were divided into four groups.

The first group (A) was composed of 10 patients on conventional low-protein diet (CLND: 0.6 g/kg/day, 35 kcal/kg/day, 700–800 mg/day of phosphorus) with oral calcium supplements (1–1.5 g/day), without any addition of phosphorus chelating agents or vitamin D metabolites; allopurinol was prescribed only when necessary. Mean blood pressure (MBP) was constantly $\leqslant$113 mm Hg and 8/10 patients were on a conventional antihypertensive treatment (diuretics, β blockers, vasodilators).

The second group (B) was composed of 11 patients who were following the same pharmacological treatment as the patients in group A but on free diet. Their MBP was well controlled.

The third group (C) included 8 patients who followed the same dietary and pharmacological treatment as the patients in group A. However, their MBP was not well enough controlled, oscillating between 117 and 123 mm Hg. This was attributed to a poor compliance with the therapy, generally due to the side effects it produced.

The fourth group (D) comprised 8 patients who were not following the prescribed CLND or who did so only irregularly and/or shortly. Also, in this group the MBP was not sufficiently controlled, as in group C.

We examined the progression of chronic renal failure as a whole in the four groups by using the serum creatinine reciprocal [14]. Compliance with the diet therapy was evaluated according to the blood urea nitrogen (BUN)/serum creatinine ratio [15]. Those patients who maintained a ratio of $\leqslant$10 at all levels of renal function were considered to have complied with the CLND.

In our second study we prospectively examined two groups of patients with different degrees of chronic renal failure. In the first group (G1), 67 patients (39 males, 28 females, age 28–59 years), with creatinine clearance (CrC) oscillating between 60 and 20 ml/min, were enrolled. The nephropathy was chronic glomerulonephritis (CGN): 40 patients; chronic pyelonephritis (CPN): 14 patients; polycystic kidney disease (PKD): 8 patients; nephroangiosclerosis (NAS): 5 patients. All patients were on a free diet and on antihypertensive treatment. The drugs used to keep blood pressure $\leqslant$160/90 mm Hg were chosen among diuretics (furosemide), β-blockers (metoprolol/athenolol), central or peripheral vasodilators (clonidine, hydralazine, prazosine), converting enzyme inhibitor (captopril). They were followed every 8 weeks with CrC and 24-hour proteinuria test (UProt) over a 12-month period. At the end of this period, a decline of renal function was assessed by a negative slope of the regression line of the values of CrC checked-up during these 12 months.

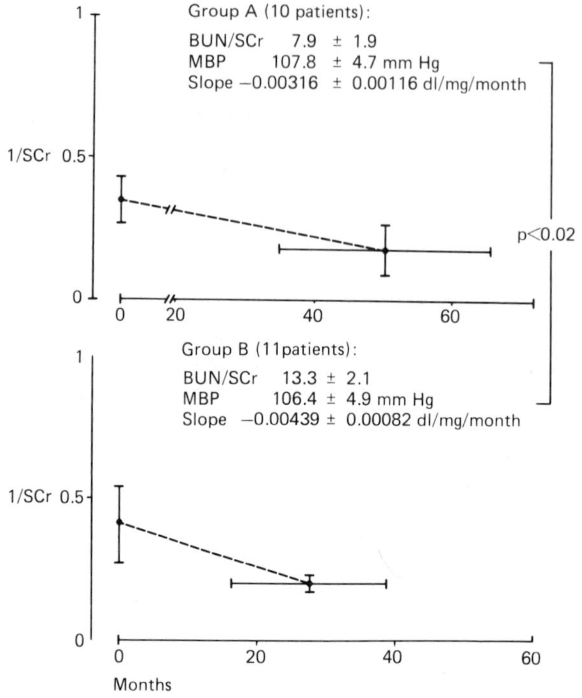

Fig. 2. Progression of chronic renal failure in group A and B patients.

The second group (G2) was composed of 51 enrolled patients (30 males and 21 females; age 22–64 years) with CrC < 20 ml/min. The nephropathy was CGN 31 patients, CPN 12 patients, PKD 5 patients, NAS 3 patients. They began CLND and antihypertensive treatment like the patients G1. In this group CrC and 24-hour proteinuria were carried out every 2 weeks. They were followed through a 3- to 12-month study period. A decline in renal function was evidenced by a negative slope of the regression line of CrC calculated from the last 5 observations performed every 2 weeks.

Results

Patients in group A, at the beginning of the 50.2 ± 15.3 month follow-up, showed serum creatinine (Crb) 2.9 ± 0.5 mg/100 ml. At the end of the follow-up, serum creatinine (Cra) was 6.7 ± 3.3 mg/100 ml with a 1/serum creatinine slope of -0.00316 ± 0.00116 dl/mg/month. The patients attended outpatient clinic check-ups 3–6 times per year. The BUN/serum creatinine ratio was stabilized at 7.9 ± 1.9. The MBP was 107.8 ± 4.7 mm Hg (fig. 2). The group B patients showed a Crb of

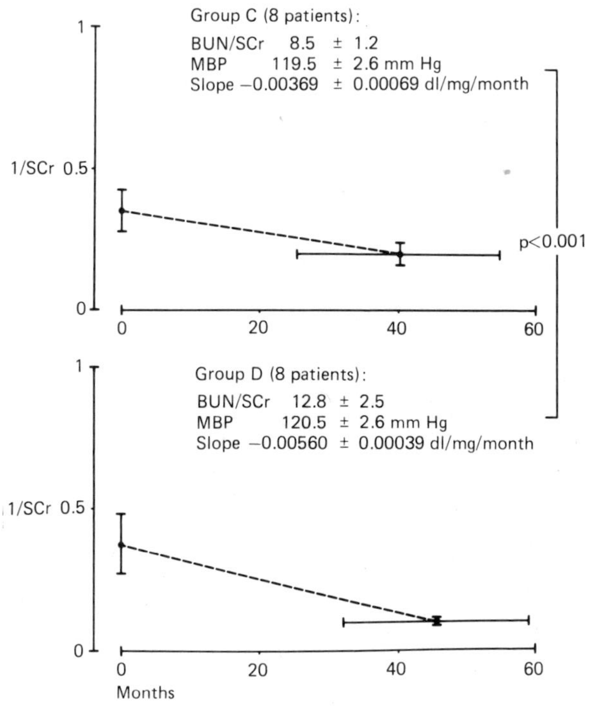

Fig. 3. Progression of chronic renal failure in group C and D patients.

2.6 ± 0.8 mg/100 ml and Cra 5.2 ± 0.9 mg/100 ml after 27.5 ± 11.1 months with a slope of − 0.00439 ± 0.00082 dl/mg/month ($p < 0.02$ vs A); checks were carried out 2–5 times per year. The BUN/serum creatinine ratio was firmly 13.3 ± 2.1. The MBP was 106.4 ± 4.9 mm Hg (fig. 2). The group C patients showed a Crb 2.9 ± 0.5 mg/100 ml and Cra 5.3 ± 1.3 mg/100 ml after 40.2 ± 14.5 months with a slope of − 0.00369 ± 0.00069 dl/mg/month (p: n.s. vs A and B); checks were carried out 3–6 times per year. The BUN/serum creatinine ratio was 8.5 ± 1.2. The MBP was 119.5 ± 2.6 mm Hg ($p < 0.001$ vs A and B) (fig. 3). The patients in group D showed a Crb of 2.9 ± 0.5 mg/100 ml, Cra 9.6 ± 1.1 mg/100 ml, follow-up 45.5 ± 13.6 months, slope of − 0.00560 ± 0.00039 dl/mg/month ($p < 0.001$ vs A and C, $p < 0.005$ vs B); MBP 120.5 ± 2.6 mm Hg ($p < 0.001$ vs A and B) (fig 3). In our second study in basal conditions the CrC and UProt of G1 and G2 were respectively 41.1 ± 7.4 and 15.6 ± 4.4 ml/min; 1,189.3 ± 855.2 and 1,563.3 ± 1,039.5 mg/24 h. The results of the prospective study are reported in figs. 4 to 7. In 18 of G1 patients CrC declined

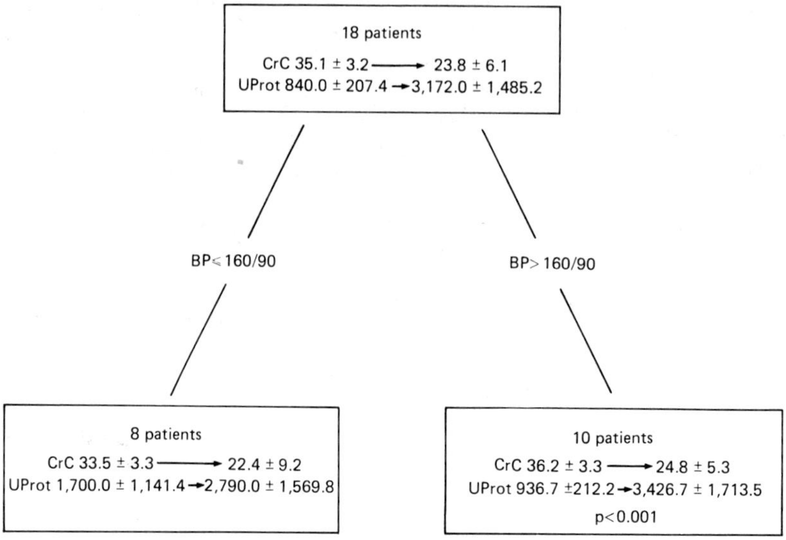

Fig. 4. Subgroups of G1 patients with declining CrC.

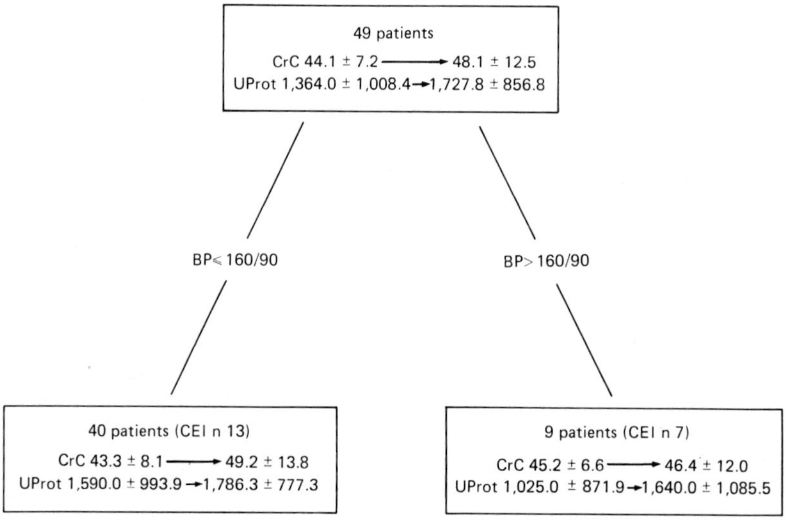

Fig. 5. Subgroups of G1 patients with stable CrC.

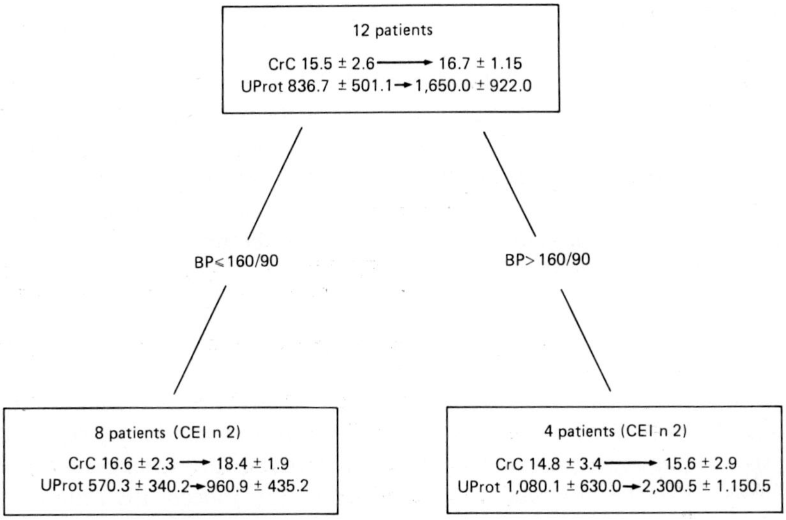

Fig. 6. Subgroups of G2 patients with stable CrC.

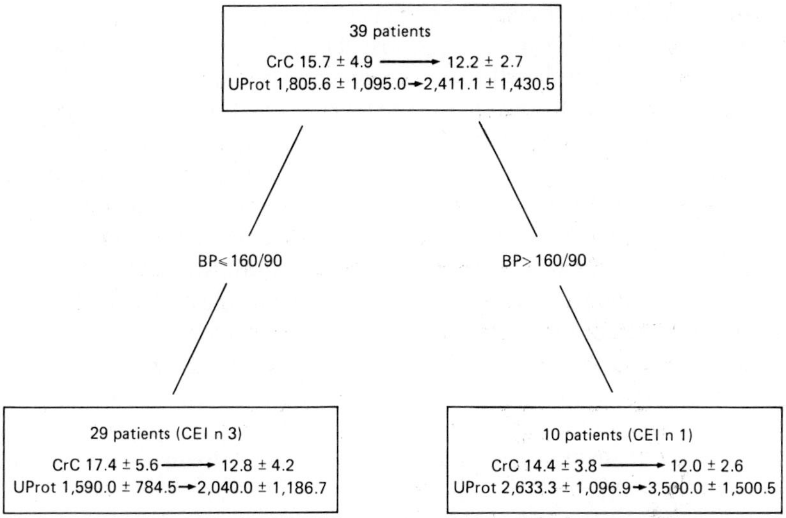

Fig. 7. Subgroups of G2 patients with declining CrC.

(fig. 4), 10 patients remained hypertensive; only in this subgroup UProt was significantly increasing. Of the 49 patients with unmodifying CrC 9 had insufficiently controlled blood pressure (7 were on Captopril treatment) (fig. 5). In G2 renal function was stable in 12 patients (fig. 6), 4 of whom were hypertensive; the glomerular filtration rate (GFR) was declining in 39 and 10 hypertensive (fig. 7); the patients on Captopril were homogeneously distributed throughout all the subgroups. In G2 a significant difference ($p < 0.05$) was observed in basal proteinuria between the two subgroups, being higher in the deteriorating one.

Discussion

As shown in the first study our data confirm that a reduction in protein intake, begun quite early in the course of chronic renal failure, slows down the progression of the disease [15]. Indeed, the progression in group A was significantly slower than in group B, blood pressure levels being equal. The protective mechanism consisting in a failure of glomerular vasodilation, is responsible for damage due to hyperfiltration [1]. A condition of glomerular equilibrium, got this way, seems to protect the surviving nephrons from the effect of systemic pressure which is not well enough controlled. Even though the group C patients had higher blood pressure values than group A, there were no significant differences in the progression of chronic renal failure. In both groups there was good compliance with the low-protein diet treatment, as evidenced by the BUN/creatinine ratios. In group D patients, however, the most damaging effect of the hypertensive state on the glomeruli reflected a poor and sporadic dietary compliance.

It seems clear from our prospective study that systemic hypertension may deteriorate renal function in patients with chronic renal failure on a free diet. In 56% of G1 patients with a progression of renal damage a hypertensive state persisted and the deteriorating renal function was linked with augmented levels of urinary proteins. This last feature can be explained by glomerular hypertension and hyperfiltration [16]. On the contrary in the patients with preserved renal function just 18% showed a poor blood pressure control; of those, 78% were on Captopril treatment. We can hypothesize that, in spite of the persistence of systemic hypertension, the possible correction of glomerular hypertension by CEI could hamper the loss of renal function greater than 20 ml/min. A renoprotective effect of CEI, from their antihypertensive action, has already been postulated [8, 12, 13, 17, 18].

Likewise, this mechanism is connected with the angiotensin production blocking action [19]. Thus CEI treatment will be characterized by a decreased intraglomerular pressure, because of the dilation of the efferent arterioles, increased renal plasma flow, unvaried glomerular filtration and possibly decreased proteinuria. Nevertheless, CEI efficacy seems to be reduced when CrC is less than 20 ml/min; it shows up from the random distribution throughout the G2 subgroups of Captopril-treated patients. On the other hand, at the same level of renal function <20 ml/min, the institution of a CLND results late to blunt the loss of surviving nephrons which otherwise appears to progress relentlessly. On these grounds proteinuria can be considered as a predictive index being significantly higher in G2 patients with declining renal function. In other words we could support the view indicating the existence of a critical point [20] in the natural history of chronic renal failure. This point seems to be at GFR ~ 20 ml/min beyond which the positive effects of dietary protein restriction and antihypertensive drugs, also working at glomerular level, are both lacking.

References

1 Brenner BM, Meyer TW, Hostetter TH: Dietary protein intake and the progressive nature of kidney disease. N Eng J Med 1982;307:652–659.

2 Brenner BM, Meyer TW: Mechanisms of progression of renal disease; in Robinson RR (ed): Proc 9th Int Congr Nephrol. New York, Springer, 1984, pp 1233–1246.

3 Baylis C, Blantz RC: Factors contributing to progression of renal disease. Int J Artif Organs 1986;9:153–158.

4 Baldwin DS, Neugarten J: Role of hypertension in the evolution of renal diseases. Contrib Nephrol 1987;54:63–76.

5 Friedlander MM, Rubinger D, Popovtzer MM: Improved renal function in patients with primary renal disease after control of severe hypertension. Am J Nephrol 1982;2:12–14.

6 Oksa H, Pasternak A, Luomala M, et al: Progression of chronic renal failure. Nephron 1983;35:31–34.

7 Anderson S, Brenner BM: Role of intraglomerular hypertension in the initiation and progression of renal disease; in Kaplan NM, Brenner BM, Laragh JH (eds): The Kidney in Hypertension. New York, Raven Press, 1987, pp 67–76.

8 Anderson S, Meyer TW, Rennke HG, et al: Control of glomerular hypertension limits glomerular injury in rats with reduced renal mass. J Clin Invest 1985;76:612–619.

9 Dworkin LD, Hostetter TH, Rennke HG, et al: Hemodynamic basis for glomerular injury in rats with desoxycorticosterone-salt hypertension. J Clin Invest 1984;73:1448–1461.

10 Raij L, Chiou X-C, Owens R, et al: Therapeutic implications of hypertension-induced glomerular injury. Am J Med 1985;79(suppl 3C):37–41.

11 Bergström J, Alvestrand A, Bucht H, et al: Progression of chronic renal failure in man is retarded with more frequent clinical follow-ups and better blood pressure control. Clin Nephrol 1986;25:1–6.

12 Anderson S, Rennke HG, Brenner BM: Therapeutic advantage of converting enzyme inhibitors in arresting progressive renal disease associated with systemic hypertension in the rat. J Clin Invest 1986;77:1993–2000.

13 Reams GP, Bauer JH: Effects of enalapril in subjects with hypertension associated with moderate to severe renal dysfunction. Arch Intern Med 1986;146:2145–2148.
14 Mitch WE, Walser M, Buffington GA, et al: A simple method of estimating progression of chronic renal failure. Lancet 1976;ii:1326–1328.
15 Kopple JD, Coburn JW: Evaluation of chronic uremia. JAMA 1974;227:41–44.
16 Rosman JB, Donker AJM, Van der Hem GK: Dietary protein restriction and the progression of renal failure. Int J Artif Organs 1986;9:77–80.
17 Meyer TW, Anderson S, Rennke HG, et al: Reversing glomerular hypertension stabilizes established glomerular injury. Kidney Int 1987;31:752–759.
18 Cappelli P, Del Rosso G, Di Paolo B, et al: Glomerular hypertension in the progression of chronic renal failure: role of low-protein diet and angiotensin converting enzyme inhibitors. Scand J Urol Nephrol 1988;(suppl 108):25–30.
19 Bauer JH, Reams GP: Renal effects of angiotensin converting enzyme inhibitors in hypertension. Am J Med 1986;81(suppl 4C):19–27.
20 Oldrizzi L, Rugiu C, Maschio G: Hypertension and progression of renal failure in patients on protein-restricted diet. Contrib Nephrol 1987;54:134–143.

Prof. Alberto Albertazzi, Institute of Nephrology, S. Camillo De Lellis University Hospital, I–66100 Chieti (Italy)

Oldrizzi L, Maschio G, Rugiu C, et al. (eds): The Progressive Nature of Renal Disease: Myths and Facts. Contrib Nephrol. Basel, Karger, 1989, vol 75, pp 177–184

Insulin in Chronic Renal Failure: Friend or Foe?

A. M. El Nahas

Department of Renal Medicine, Northern General Hospital, Sheffield, England, UK

During the course of chronic renal failure (CRF) many endocrine and metabolic disturbances take place [1]. It has recently been suggested that some of these hormonal and metabolic alterations may play a major role in the progression of the underlying renal scarring process [2]. In this review, I will concentrate on the contribution of insulin and insulin-like growth factor-I (IGF-I)/somatomedin-C to the metabolic profile of chronic uraemia and explore their possible role in the pathogenesis of renal scarring.

Insulin and IGF-I share considerable structural and biological similarities [3]. These include their metabolic and growth-promoting effects [3]. In CRF the basal immunoreactive levels of insulin [4] and IGF-I [5] are often raised. Circulating inhibitors of their biological activities have been detected in the serum of patients with CRF [6–8]. Consequently, insulin resistance is universal in these patients. Such resistance has considerable repercussions on the metabolism of carbohydrates, protein and lipids in uraemia.

Role of Insulin Resistance in the Pathophysiology of the Abnormal Metabolism of Chronic Uraemia

Carbohydrate Metabolism in Chronic Renal Failure

In chronic uraemia, carbohydrate metabolism is affected by the interplay of many hormones. Of all these, the peripheral resistance to the action of insulin, invariably present in CRF, plays a preponderant role [1]. The expression of hyperglycaemia or glucose intolerance in chronic uraemia depends on the balance between such peripheral resistance and the capacity of the pancreatic islet β-cells to increase their insulin secretion [1]. In CRF, such secretion is suppressed by secondary hyperparathyroidism [9] as well as the deficiency in 1,25-vitamin D_3 [10]. Finally, the increase in serum cortisol, growth hormone and glucagon levels in CRF is also likely to contribute to the observed carbohydrate intolerance [1].

Protein Metabolism in Chronic Renal Failure

Patients with CRF are often wasted and suffer from a decrease in lean body mass. Protein metabolism in CRF depends on the overall balance between protein synthesis and degradation. In CRF, abnormalities of protein metabolism are likely to be multifactorial [11]. However, it is likely that the decreased protein synthesis and the increased muscle protein breakdown are the most important causes of protein catabolism in chronic uraemia.

Insulin plays a major role in the regulation of protein synthesis and metabolism. In acute uraemia, the observed decreased protein synthesis is directly linked to the abnormalities in insulin-stimulated glucose metabolism [12]. The effects of insulin resistance on protein metabolism in CRF remain to be determined. As abnormal insulin action is likely to contribute to the excessive muscle protein breakdown in CRF. Recent observations imply that hyperglucagonaemia accelerates protein catabolism in the presence of insulin deficiency [13]. Other factors that contribute to the excessive muscle proteolysis in CRF include metabolic acidosis and hypercorticism [14].

Lipid Metabolism in Chronic Renal Failure

The majority of patients with CRF display various degrees of hyperlipidaemia. Such hyperlipidaemia, as in the case of protein metabolism, is likely to be the reflection of the overall balance between lipid synthesis and breakdown.

As with carbohydrate and protein metabolisms, insulin plays an important role in the pathogenesis of the hyperlipidaemia of CRF. Insulin resistance-induced hyperglycaemia increases hepatic production of triglycerides [15]. Hyperinsulinaemia can also stimulate triglyceride synthesis. However, in CRF, the pathogenesis of hyperlipidaemia seems to depend predominantly on a decreased breakdown of triglyceride-rich particles. Such a breakdown is normally regulated by both hepatic lipase and post-heparin lipoprotein lipase activities. These are affected by changes in apoproteins and LCAT activity in CRF [1]. Insulin is also a well-known regulator of lipoprotein lipase activity, and resistance to its action contributes to the decreased activity of this enzyme in uraemia [16].

Mechanism of Insulin Resistance in Uraemia

Insulin and IGF-I exert their biological effects through two separate receptors [3]. The biological activities of these polypeptides are initiated through their binding to a glycoprotein receptor that consists of two subunits. The α-subunit binds the hormone, whereas the β-subunit is an insulin-sensitive tyrosine-specific protein kinase. The activation of the β-subunit and its insulin-mediated phosphorylation initiate the expression of the cellular effects of insulin [3].

Some degree of insulin resistance is an early and universal finding in uraemia. It is currently thought that a small molecular weight circulating peptide, normally excreted by the kidneys, accumulates in CRF and inhibits insulin action [6]. The inhibition of insulin action takes place at a post-receptor, post-tyrosine kinase level of the molecular action of insulin [8]. It has been postulated that cell membrane phospholipids mediate the intracellular effects of insulin [17]. It is tempting to speculate that changes in these cellular constituents, known to take place in CRF [18], contribute to the insulin resistance of uraemia.

In this review, I would like to postulate that the hyperinsulinaemia and increased IGF-I observed in CRF, whilst beneficial in overcoming the peripheral insulin resistance of uraemia, contribute to the acceleration of glomerular scarring in the presence of hyperglycaemia and hyperlipidaemia.

Role of Insulin in the Development of Renal Scarring

Stages of Glomerular Scarring

It is likely that glomerular scarring proceeds within individual glomeruli through a succession of stages. Following an acute reduction in functional renal mass, an early stage (I) of compensatory glomerular hypertrophy and hyperfunction takes place in the glomeruli spared by the initial insult [19]. The contribution of these adaptive changes to the progression of glomerulosclerosis (GS) remains the subject of controversy. The second stage (II) of glomerular scarring is characterized by damage to glomerular cells. This can result from either the initial injury or the secondary glomerular adaptive adjustments. During this stage, damage to the glomerular endothelium is likely to attract platelets and monocytes into scarred glomeruli. These would interact with glomerular cells to initiate GS.

During this stage (III), glomerular scarring bears striking similarities to the process of large vessel atherosclerosis [2, 20]. It is characterized by glomerular infiltration by platelets and monocytes, proliferation of smooth muscle-like mesangial cells and the deposition within the glomeruli of plasma proteins and lipids. This culminates in glomerular microthrombosis and hyalinosis with obliteration of the glomerular capillary tuft. The final stage (IV) of GS is that of progressive glomerular fibrosis leading to end-stage renal failure.

Role of Insulin and IGF-I in Glomerulosclerosis

Both insulin and IGF-I could, in theory, be involved in every step of the development of GS. During the early stage of adaptive renal growth an increase in the kidney content of IGF-I takes place in rats following renal ablation [21] and in those with diabetic nephropathy [22]. Glomerular hypertrophy is also known to take place in transgenic mice with high circulating levels of IGF-I [23]. Whilst a causal relationship between the rise in renal IGF-I and renal hypertrophy remains to be established, experimental evidence suggests an effect of IGF-I and insulin on renal growth. Both peptides are capable of stimulating the proliferation of renal cells in vitro [24, 25]. IGF-I may also mediate the adaptive glomerular haemodynamic changes [26].

During stage II of glomerular scarring, insulin and IGF-I could interact with endothelial and mesangial cells and contribute to glomerular cellular injury. Vascular endothelium has receptors for IGF-I whereas mesangial cells, like their smooth-muscle counterpart, have receptors for both insulin and IGF-I [25]. IGF-I have been implicated in the mitotic effect of human diabetic serum on endothelial cells [27]. IGF-I can also stimulate the binding of lipids to vascular endothelium.

IGF-I, and to a lesser extent insulin, are capable of stimulating the invitro proliferation of mesangial cells [25]. Insulin enhances the uptake of lipids by smooth muscle cells [28]. A similar effect on mesangial cells is anticipated in CRF in the presence of hyperlipidemia. Lipids accumulation within mesangial cells is characteristic of scarred glomeruli [29]. This may contribute to mesangial dysfunction and accelerate GS. At this stage, IGF-I may also lead to an increase in extracellular matrix (ECM) formation as it stimulates the production of proteoglycans by microvascular endothelium [30]. This, together with the stimulatory effect of hyperglycaemia on endothelial production of collagen [31], would lead to the expansion of glomerular ECM. Mesangial proliferation and ECM expansion are common features of early glomerular scarring.

During stage III of GS, platelets and monocytes infiltrate the glomeruli. Insulin stimulates the uptake of lipids by monocytes [32]. This could accelerate their transformation to foam cells. Many such foam cells infiltrate scarred glomeruli [29]. The subsequent release by these lipid-laden macrophages of oxidized lipids could lead to further GS. Insulin has been implicated in the pathogenesis of atherosclerosis (ATS) [33]. In view of the pathophysiological similarities between ATS and GS, it is tempting to speculate that it plays an equally important role in the pathogenesis of the latter.

Finally, during the last stage (IV) of glomerular scarring, fibroblasts infiltrate scarred glomeruli. During this stage, the release by platelets and monocytes of factors such as PDGF, fibroblast growth factor and macrophage growth factor can stimulate the production of IGF-I by these fibroblasts [34]. This would initiate further fibrosis, as IGF-I itself is a potent fibroblast mitogen [35]. Other GF, such as transforming growth factor-β, can also stimulate glomerular collagen production and lead to their fibrosis [36].

Insulin Resistance and Systemic Hypertension

Systemic hypertension often precedes the development of CRF in patients with chronic nephropathies. Its onset accelerates the decline in renal function. Hyperinsulinaemia and insulin resistance have been linked to the development of systemic hypertension [37]. Insulin resistance in hypertension could be caused by the changes in cell membrane phospholipids known to take place in this condition [38]. As similar changes have recently been reported in CRF [18], these may underly both the development of insulin resistance and the hypertension often associated with chronic nephropathies. Changes in plasma membrane lipids and the associated insulin resistance can contribute to the development of hypertension through changes in the intracellular content of cations (sodium/calcium) [18].

In summary, it is conceivable that hyperinsulinaemia and a raised IGF-I may, in the presence of hyperglycaemia and hyperlipidaemia, contribute to the progression of renal scarring. Hyperinsulinaemia may also play a role in the development of systemic hypertension in patients with CRF.

Clinical and Therapeutic Implications

A unifying hypothesis, linking insulin resistance to the development of metabolic derangements, hypertension and the progression of renal scarring in CRF, could have important therapeutic implications. An improvement in the underlying insulin resistance by dietary or pharmacological means would not only correct the metabolic derangements but also attenuate the hypertension and GS of CRF. Such an assumption is supported by the fact that many therapeutic interventions known to improve insulin resistance are of potential benefit in the management of progressive CRF. For instance, increased physical activity is known to increase tissue sensitivity to insulin. Exercise training also improves hyperlipidaemia and prevents progressive GS in experimental animals [39].

Similarly, diets low in protein [40] and those supplemented with polyunsaturated fat reduce insulin resistance [41]. They also correct hyperlipidaemia, reduce hypertension and slow the progression of experimental CRF [42].

Further studies are required to establish the link between the potential beneficial effects of these dietary interventions in CRF and their effect on insulin resistance. In the meanwhile, in the presence of some resistance to their metabolic effects, insulin and IGF-I are likely to be foes rather than friends.

References

1 Eknoyan G: Effects of renal insufficiency on nutrient metabolism and endocrine function; in Mitch WE, Klahr S (eds): Nutrition and the kidney. Boston, Little, Brown, 1988, pp 29–58.

2 El Nahas AM: Glomerulosclerosis: A form of atherosclerosis; in Davison AM (ed): Nephrology. London, Ballière-Tindall, 1988, vol II, pp 1206–1218.

3 Kahn CR: The molecular mechanism of insulin action. Annu Rev Med 1985;36:429–451.

4 De Fronzo RA: Pathogenesis of glucose intolerance in uraemia. Metabolism 1978;27(suppl 2):1866–18880.

5 Powell DR, Rosefeld RE, Sperry JB, et al: Serum concentrations of insulin-like growth factor I, IGF-2 and unsaturated somatomedin carrier proteins in children with chronic renal failure. Am J Kidney Dis 1987;10:287–292.

6 McCaleb ML, Izzo MS, Lockwood DH: Characterization and partial purification of a factor from uremic human serum that induces insulin resistance. J Clin Invest 1985;75:391–396.

7 Phillips LS, Fusco AC, Unterman TG, et al: Somatomedin inhibitor in uremia. J Clin Endocrinol Metab 1984;59:764–772.

8 Cecchin F, Ittoop O, Sinha MK, et al: Insulin resistance in uremia: insulin receptor kinase activity in liver and muscle from chronic uremic rats. Am J Physiol 1988;254:E394–E401.

9 Mak RHK, Bettinelli A, Turner L, et al: The influence of hyperparathyroidism on glucose metabolism in uremia. J Clin Endocrinol Metab 1985;60:229–233.

10 Mak RHK: Intravenous 1,25-vitamin D_3 restores glucose tolerance, increases insulin secretion and corrects insulin resistance in uremic patients on hemodialysis. 5th Int Congr Nutr Metabolism in Renal Disease, Strasbourg, 1988, abstr 115.

11 Mitch WE: Uremia and the control of protein metabolism. Nephron 1988;49:89–93.

12 May RC, Clark AS, Goheer A, et al: Identification of specific defects in insulin-mediated muscle metabolism in acute uremia. Kidney Int 1985;28:490–497.

13 Nair KS, Halliday D, Matthews DE, et al: Hyperglucagonemia during insulin deficiency accelerates protein catabolism. Am J Physiol 1987;253:E208–213.

14 May RC, Kelly RA, Mitch WE: Metabolic acidosis stimulates protein degradation in rat muscle by a glucocorticoid-dependent mechanism. J Clin Invest 1986;77:614–621.

15 Sanfelippo ML, Swenson RS, Reaven GM: Response of plasma triglycerides to dietary change in patients on haemodialysis. Kidney Int 1978;14:180–184.

16 Ibels LS, Reardon MF, Nestel PJ: Plasma post-heparin lipolytic activity and triglyceride clearance in uremic and haemodialysis patients and renal allograft recipients. J Lab Clin Med 1976;87:648–652.

17 Saltiel AR, Cuatrecasas P: In search of a second messenger for insulin. Am J Physiol 1988;255:C1–C11.

18 Mich WE, Druml W: Mechanisms of protein catabolism in chronic renal failure: the influence of acid-base status. 5th Int Congr Nutr Renal Metabolism, Strasbourg, 1988, abstr 121.
19 Hostetter TH, Olson JL, Rennke HG, et al: Hyperfiltration in remnant nephrons: a potentially adverse response to renal ablation. Am J Physiol 1981;241:F85–F93.
20 Diamond JR, Karnovsky MJ: Focal and segmental glomerulosclerosis: Analogies to atherosclerosis. Kidney Int 1988;33:917–924.
21 Fagin JA, Melmed S: Relative increase in insulin-like growth factor I messenger ribonucleic acid levels in compensatory renal hypertrophy. Endocrinology 1987;12:718–721.
22 Flyvbjerg A, Thorlacius-Ussing O, Naeraa R, et al: Kidney tissue somatomedin C and initial renal growth in diabetic and uninephrectomised rats. Diabetologia 1988;31:310–314.
23 Doi T, Striker LJ, Quaife C, et al: Progressive glomerulosclerosis develops in transgenic mice chronically expressing growth hormone and growth hormone releasing factor but not those expressing insulin-like growth factor-1. Am J Pathol 1988;131:398–403.
24 Fine LG, Badie-Dezfouly B, Lowe AG: Stimulation of Na/H antiport is an early event in hypertrophy of renal proximal tubular cells. Proc Natl Acad Sci USA 1985;82:1736–1740.
25 Conti FG, Striker CJ, Lesniak MA, et al: Studies on binding and mitogenic effect of insulin and insulin-like growth factor I in glomerular mesangial cells. Endocrinology 1988;122:2788–2795.
26 Hirschberg R, Kopple JD: Growth hormone and IGF-I modulate renal function. Kidney Int 1989;35:312A.
27 Petty RG, Pearson JD, Morgan DML: Simulation of endothelial cell growth by sera from diabetic patients with retinopathy. Lancet 1988;i:208–211.
28 Young IR, Stout RW: Effects of insulin and glucose in the cells of the arterial wall: interaction of insulin with dibutyryl cyclic AMP and low-density lipoprotein in arterial cells. Diabète Métab 1987;13:301–306.
29 Grond J, Van Goor H, Erkelens DW, et al: Glomerular sclerotic lesions in the rat. Virchows Arch [Cell Pathol] 1980;51:521–524.
30 Bar RS, Dake BL, Stueck S: Stimulation of proteoglycans by IGF-I and II in microvessel and large endothelial cells. Am J Physiol 1987;253:E21–E27.
31 Cagliero E, Maiello M, Boeri D, et al: Increased expression of basement membrane components in human endothelial cells cultured in high glucose. J Clin Invest 1988;82:735–738.
32 Krone W, Greten H: Evidence for post-transcriptional regulation by insulin of 3-hydroxy-3-methylglutaryl coenzyme A reductase and sterol synthesis in human mononuclear leucocytes. Diabetologia 1984;26:366–369.
33 Stout RW: Insulin and atheroma – an update. Lancet 1987;i:1077–1079.
34 Clemmons DR: Multiple hormones stimulate the production of somatomedin by cultured human fibroblasts. J Clin Endocrinol Metab 1984;58:850–856.
35 Conover CA, Dollar LA, Hintz RL, et al: IGF-I/SMC and glucocorticoids synergistically regulate mitosis in competent human fibroblasts. J Cell Physiol 1983;116:191–197.
36 McNamara MM, Ballerman BJ: Influence of transforming growth factor-β and glomerular endothelial cell-conditioned medium on mesangial cell matrix synthesis. Kidney Int 1989;35:432.
37 Modan M, Halkin H, Almog E, et al: Hyperinsulinemia. A link between hypertension, obesity and glucose intolerance. J Clin Invest 1985;75:809–817.

38 Bing RF, Heagerty AM, Thurston H, et al: Ion transport in hypertension: are changes in the cell membrane responsible? Clin Sci 1986;71:225–230.
39 Heifets M, Davis TA, Tegtmeyer E, et al: Exercise training ameliorates progressive renal disease in rats with subtotal nephrectomy. Kidney Int 1987;32:815–820.
40 Mak RHK, Turner C, Thompson T, et al: Glucose metabolism in children with uremia: Effect of dietary phosphate and protein. Kidney Int 1987;32:S206–S209.
41 Vanhouny GV: Conclusions and recommendations of the symposium on 'dietary fibers in health and disease'. Am J Clin Nutr 1982;35:152–156.
42 El Nahas AM: Management of progressive renal failure: the role of dietary manipulations. Postgrad Med J 1988;63:611–615.

Dr. A. M. El Nahas, Northern General Hospital,
Herries Road, GB-Sheffield S5 7AU (UK)

Oldrizzi L, Maschio G, Rugiu C, et al. (eds): The Progressive Nature of Renal Disease: Myths and Facts. Contrib Nephrol. Basel, Karger, 1989, vol 75, pp 185–193

Amino Acid Imbalance in Patients with Chronic Renal Failure

Alberto Tizianello, Giacomo Deferrari, Giacomo Garibotto, Cristina Robaudo, Stefano Saffioti, Roberto Pontremoli

Istituto Scientifico di Medicina Interna, Sections of Nephrology and Clinical Methodology, University of Genoa, Italy

It is assumed that a healthy 70-kg adult man requires an intake of about 50 g/day of protein in order to replace his daily protein waste and so to maintain homeostasis of body protein. Such an amount is actually small when it is compared with that recycled in endogenous protein turnover; in fact, every day about 300 g of protein, mainly muscle protein, are degraded and nearly 80% of the amino acids (AA) so released are reutilized for new protein synthesis. The free AA pool can be considered a connecting link between exogenous protein metabolism and endogenous protein turnover [1]. AA levels in blood represent the result of all events affecting total body AA flow. Thus, in the postabsorptive state, that is after a 12- to 14-hour overnight fast, blood AA levels reflect mainly endogenous protein turnover. Actually, in the postabsorptive state AA are released into the circulation from muscle and also kidney, while splanchnic organs, kidney and brain utilize them [2].

Blood Amino Acid Levels in the Postabsorptive State

Abnormalities in blood AA levels occurring in patients with chronic renal failure (CRF) have been recognized for a long time [3, 4]. However, difficulties in understanding the meaning of these alterations have been found, mainly owing to the similarities with the blood AA profile observed in exogenous malnutrition [5]. Malnutrition, on the other hand, often occurs in patients with advanced uremia or treated with incorrect diets [5]. More recently, it has become clear that many abnormalities in the blood AA profile are induced by renal failure per se [3, 6].

Studies have been carried out in our laboratory with the purpose of defining abnormalities in blood AA typical in CRF. Only patients with CRF before the uremic stage and on an unrestricted diet were evaluated.

Table 1. Arterial levels of AA in whole blood in 25 patients with CRF and in 32 controls studied in the postabsorptive state[a]

	AA levels, μmol/liter		
	controls	CRF[b]	p[c]
Taurine	189.1 ± 6.8	203.2 ± 8.6	n.s.[d]
Aspartate	124.9 ± 6.7	82.7 ± 7.8	<0.001
Threonine	103.8 ± 3.2	90.2 ± 3.3	<0.005
Serine	110.9 ± 3.1	87.3 ± 2.6	<0.001
Glutamate[e]	141.4 ± 3.6	132.2 ± 4.6	n.s.
Glutamine[e]	520.5 ± 11.0	478.0 ± 15.0	n.s.
Proline	134.0 ± 5.6	229.0 ± 12.8	<0.001
Glycine	242.5 ± 6.9	259.0 ± 10.4	n.s.
Alanine	216.5 ± 6.2	211.8 ± 6.6	n.s.
Citrulline	30.0 ± 0.9	61.9 ± 2.4	<0.001
Valine	181.7 ± 5.0	155.4 ± 4.9	<0.001
Isoleucine	49.9 ± 1.4	46.9 ± 1.9	n.s.
Leucine	96.3 ± 2.5	88.1 ± 4.1	n.s.
Tyrosine	41.7 ± 1.2	31.6 ± 1.8	<0.001
Phenylalanine	38.2 ± 0.8	38.2 ± 1.0	n.s.
Ornithine	74.1 ± 2.3	77.9 ± 3.1	n.s.
Lysine	141.6 ± 3.2	137.5 ± 4.9	n.s.
Histidine	63.3 ± 1.4	80.2 ± 2.9	<0.001
Arginine	66.2 ± 1.6	61.3 ± 2.9	n.s.
Cyst(e)ine	49.3 ± 2.0	70.2 ± 2.6	<0.001
Triptophan	47.4 ± 3.0	33.0 ± 2.8	<0.005

[a] Data are expressed as mean ± SEM. Adapted from Tizianello et al. [6–8, 15] and Deferrari et al. [9, 10, 18, 19].
[b] In the 13 patients with GFR < 20 ml/min citrulline, aspartate, tyrosine, leucine, glutamine, arginine and glutamate became significantly altered or even more than in the 12 patients with GFR > 20 ml/min.
[c] Significance of difference between patients with CRF and controls.
[d] Not significant.
[e] Enzymatically determined.

AA assays were carried out in whole blood instead of plasma, taking into consideration the role played by blood cells in AA transport; in addition, arterial blood as opposed to venous blood was used for analyses, because the AA profile obtained from the former is not affected by the metabolism of the drained organs and tissues. Twenty-five patients with CRF (GFR 20 ± 2 ml/min · 1.73 m^2) and 32 normal controls well matched with regard to sex and body weight were studied in the postabsorptive state and the blood AA profile of the two groups compared (table 1). Typical alterations in patients are higher levels of citrulline, proline, cyst(e)ine and histidine, and lower levels of aspartate, total tryptophan, tyrosine, serine, valine, and threonine. In patients with more severe renal failure (GFR < 20 ml/min · 1.73 m^2) leucine, glutamine, arginine and glutamate are also decreased. Similar alterations have been observed by other groups in patients with CRF selected according to the above-reported criteria, as reviewed elsewhere [6]. In addition, 1- and 3-methylhistidine are also increased [6]. In conclusion, changes in blood AA profile occur in well-nourished patients with relatively preserved renal function and therefore are likely caused by renal failure per se.

Amino Acid Exchange Across the Organs in the Postabsorptive State

In order to elucidate the mechanisms responsible for these abnormalities, arterial-venous differences for AA and blood flow across the major organs involved in their metabolism were measured. In this way AA exchanges across the organs can be expressed as rates of release or uptake.

Several abnormalities have been detected. AA metabolism in peripheral tissues, of which muscle is the largest component, was evaluated by measuring AA exchange across the leg. Results obtained demonstrate that the release of valine and leucine from the leg is decreased in patients; such a decrease is likely responsible for the lower blood levels of these AA observed in patients [6, 9]. In addition, net muscle proteolysis is not increased in patients with moderate CRF, as can be deduced from AA release from peripheral tissues. Actually, the release of total AA, including alanine and glutamine, which account for more than 50% of total AA release, and the release of tyrosine, phenylalanine and lysine, which are neither synthesized nor catabolized by muscle, are similar in patients and controls [6, 8, 9]. It has been supposed that the selective abnormalities in muscle branched-chain AA (BCAA) metabolism reflect an increased degradation [7] promoted by the impaired glucose utilization [10, 11] and/or metabolic acidosis [12].

The importance of the human kidney in the AA metabolism and in their homeostasis is emphasized by observations obtained in our laboratory [4, 13, 14]. In the postabsorptive state the kidney is the only source for circulating serine, while it shares the release of tyrosine into the systemic circulation almost equally with muscle. Patients with CRF show a low renal release of serine and tyrosine; the lower the release of these AA, the lower are their arterial levels [8, 13]. In addition, in patients the renal release of arginine is also decreased, likely owing to a decreased utilization of its precursor, citrulline [8, 13]. Actually, this last AA as well as proline are utilized by the diseased kidney in lower amounts, probably accounting for the higher arterial levels of these AA [8, 13]. Finally, also the renal uptake of glutamine is markedly decreased in patients. In this condition renal ammonia production must derive from substrates different from glutamine supplied by the arterial blood [8, 13]. In postabsorptive patients with CRF abnormalities in circulating AA affect AA uptake by splanchnic organs [8, 10, 15] which are the major site for AA utilization [2]. Thus, in patients, splanchnic organs take up larger amounts of proline and histidine which are increased in arterial blood; significant correlations between arterial levels of these AA and their splanchnic uptake were found [8, 15]. These data suggest that the high arterial levels of these AA promote their abnormal splanchnic uptake. Furthermore, in patients the uptake of serine and glutamine are lower than in controls. The occurrence of a decreased fractional extraction of these AA by the splanchnic organs suggests that intrinsic metabolic defects, more than alterations in circulating AA levels, are responsible for the decreased utilization [8, 15]. Recently, in a small group of patients the uptake of alanine was greater [16]. It is interesting that splanchnic uptake of total glycogenic AA is similar to controls as well as glucose release into the hepatic veins [10, 11]. These results further support the assumption that hepatic gluconeogenesis is not increased in CRF [6, 10].

Also cerebral AA metabolism is markedly affected by changes in the circulating AA profile observed in postabsorptive patients with CRF. It is well known that AA levels in arterial blood, besides cerebral blood flow and blood-brain barrier permeability, are a major factor in the regulation of AA entry into the brain [17]. On the basis of these assumptions, abnormalities in cerebral AA uptake could be expected in CRF. Actually, when exchanges of AA across the brain were measured, it was observed that in renal patients the cerebral uptake of valine, glutamine and isoleucine is reduced, while that of glycine and cyst(e)ine is enhanced [18–20]. The altered uptake of valine, glycine and cyst(e)ine is caused by the abnormal arterial levels of these AA and those which compete for the same transport system. As for glutamine and isoleucine, an intrinsic defect in the cerebral transport and/or metabolism of these AA has been supposed [4, 18].

In conclusion, CRF precociously promotes a number of abnormalities in AA metabolism reflected by an altered circulating AA profile. For some AA these alterations can be accounted for by abnormalities in AA exchange across the organs. At the same time, changes in arterial AA levels modify AA uptake by the utilizing organs. All the data indicate the existence of an abnormal endogenous protein turnover occurring early in CRF.

Studies in the Protein-Fed State

Both the amount and quality of protein in diets for patients with CRF are crucial in order to ensure nitrogen balance, nutritional status as well as to reduce uremic toxicity and, probably, to slow down the progression of renal failure [5]. Despite these well-accepted premises, only recently attention has been paid to the events dealing with nitrogen compound metabolism in patients with CRF after the ingestion of a protein meal. Studies in which intravenous infusion of AA was used cannot shed light on this issue. In fact, metabolism of ingested protein across the splanchnic organs is essential for the actual postprandial flow of nutrients from hepatic veins into the systemic circulation and, accordingly, for nitrogen repletion of various organs and tissues [21].

Studies on the postprandial fate of ingested protein were performed in our laboratory by giving a grilled lean beef steak (4 g/kg body weight) to patients with CRF and normal controls. Criteria in the selection of patients and controls were the same as those reported above. Arterial blood samples were repeatedly taken before and during 270 min after the meal, and arterial AA levels measured [22, 23]. Arterial levels of many AA increase greatly for a long time after the protein meal in both groups. However, in patients, marked alterations in postprandial arterial levels of many AA are found (fig. 1). After the protein meal total nonessential AA (NEAA) increase much more than in normal subjects (+52%, $p < 0.025$) as a consequence of an exaggerated and prolonged increase in arterial levels of proline, glutamine, glycine, serine, cyst(e)ine and alanine. On the contrary, total essential AA (EAA) increase to the same extent as in normal subjects; however, threonine, phenylalanine and histidine levels increase more than in controls, whereas triptophan rises less than in controls. To conclude, in patients with CRF after protein ingestion the arterial profile of AA is markedly imbalanced owing to abnormalities in postprandial increments in blood AA levels. These abnormalities overlap with those observed in the postabsorptive state. It is noteworthy that only serine levels are corrected by the ingestion of a protein meal [22, 23].

In order to elucidate the factors responsible for this imbalance, we have evaluated the effects of the ingestion of an AA mixture (0.8 g/kg body weight), simulating an animal protein meal, on AA exchange across splanchnic organs. After the ingestion of the AA mixture we found a set of abnormalities in arterial levels of AA quite similar to those we observed after the steak ingestion [24, 25].

It is known that after a protein meal, in normal subjects most NEAA are captured by splanchnic organs, while the essential ones, mainly BCAA, escape into hepatic veins [16, 21]. Thus, arterial levels of many AA increase

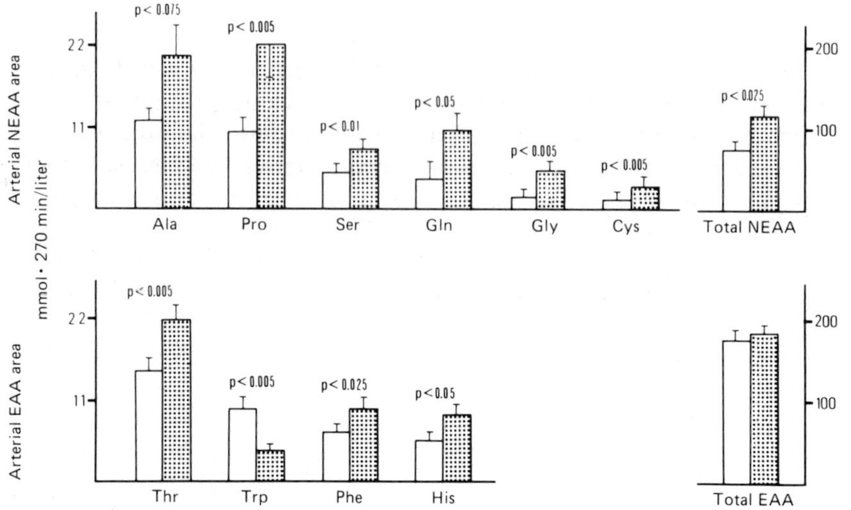

Fig. 1. Major abnormalities in AA metabolism after a protein meal in patients with CRF. Results are expressed as areas under the curves of increments in arterial levels of AA (mean ± SEM) during 270 min following the ingestion of a beef steak in 7 patients with CRF (dotted columns) and in 7 controls (blank columns).

accordingly to a profile arranged mainly by splanchnic metabolism [16, 21]. So arranged, AA are utilized by extrasplanchnic organs for nitrogen repletion.

In patients with CRF after AA ingestion, NEAA metabolism shows the most marked alterations. In fact, contrarily to what happens in controls, an augmented and prolonged splanchnic escape of proline, alanine, serine, glycine and glutamate is observed [16]. Such an escape is associated with abnormal elevations in the arterial levels of the same AA [24]. Glutamine exhibits a unique behavior. This AA, normally extracted by splanchnic organs in the postprandial period, shows a splanchnic uptake significantly greater in patients. Nevertheless, postprandial arterial levels of glutamine are markedly increased [16, 24]. These results strongly support the exclusive role of extrasplanchnic tissues in increasing arterial glutamine levels after AA ingestion. Also some EAA, namely isoleucine, threonine, phenylalanine and histidine, escape from splanchnic organs in greater amounts than in controls [16]; at the same time the last three AA show an abnormal increase in their arterial levels [24]. In CRF the splanchnic escape of BCAA is normal; it is important to note that while in controls these AA are 50% of the total AA splanchnic escape, in patients they are only 37%, owing to their dilution by the exaggerated escape of many other AA [16]. In accordance with these data, the increase in BCAA relative to total AA is lower in arterial blood [24]. When total EAA and total NEAA are considered, it appears that their splanchnic escape is 67 and 135% increased, respectively, in patients in comparison to controls, again indicating that the preeminent derangement in postprandial splanchnic metabolism regards NEAA [16].

Taken together, these results demonstrate that in CRF metabolism of ingested protein is abnormal, mainly as a consequence of an altered splanchnic metabolism involving several AA. However, biochemical derangements underlying these alterations are poorly understood. Postprandial increments in insulin levels in patients are similar to those observed in control subjects [16, 24]; thus postprandial abnormalities in AA levels do not depend on an impaired insulin availability. We have raised the hypothesis that an altered transport into hepatocytes through system A could be responsible for the exaggerated splanchnic escape of alanine, glycine, serine, proline and threonine [16]. As for phenylalanine, cyst(e)ine and tryptophan an altered hepatic metabolism can be supposed [6, 16].

Conclusions

So far the consequences of abnormalities in AA metabolism in both the postabsorptive and protein-fed state are poorly understood. It is however reasonable to suppose that, from a general point of view, the imbalance in arterial AA profile can be harmful by itself if, as is commonly asserted, an appropriate profile of AA must be supplied to cells at the same time [26, 27]. If whole organs are taken into consideration, research reported here demonstrates that the altered blood AA profile is responsible for the abnormalities in cerebral AA uptake occurring in the postabsorptive state [18, 20] and, likely, after a protein meal [22]; cerebral neurotransmitter and protein synthesis, which are dependent on the supply of precursor AA, may be altered. In addition, blood AA imbalance may be harmful for muscle tissue mainly in the postprandial period, when its nitrogen balance is reversed to a positive one and protein pools are restored. Finally, AA imbalance may be injurious also to the kidney because the exaggerated postprandial supply of NEAA to this organ may accelerate the progression of renal insufficiency according to the hyperfiltration hypothesis [28] and/or by toxic effects on renal tissues.

In conclusion, in patients with CRF before the uremic stage, blood AA profile and interorgan flow of AA are altered both in the postabsorptive state and after protein ingestion. These alterations are important hallmarks of derangements in the nitrogen compound metabolism taking place rather precociously in CRF and likely caused by this pathological condition per se. Both endogenous protein turnover and ingested protein metabolism are altered. The biochemical bases of these abnormalities as well as their clinical consequences have to be investigated. We think that abnormalities in the circulating AA profile deserve more attention in the clinical evaluation of patients with CRF and can be usefully taken into consideration in designing the nutritional treatment and in prescribing formulae of AA supplements for patients.

Acknowledgements

This study was supported by grants from the Ministero della Pubblica Istruzione (assegnazione per la Ricerca scientifica 40 and 60%) and by grants from the Consiglio Nazionale delle Ricerche (Terapia sostitutiva nelle gravi insufficienze d'organo and Progetto Finalizzato di Medicina Preventiva, Sp 4, Obiettivo 47b).

The authors wish to thank Mr. M. Bruzzone and Mrs. M.R. Sala for their excellent technical assistance, and Mrs. F. Tincani for preparation of the manuscript and figure.

References

1 Waterlow JC: Protein turnover with special reference to man. Q J Exp Physiol 1984;69:409–438.

2 Felig P: Amino acid metabolism in man. Annu Rev Biochem 1975;44:933–955.

3 Kopple JD: Amino acid metabolism in chronic renal failure; in Blackburn GL, Grant JP, Young VR, Wright J (eds): Amino Acid Metabolism and Medical Applications. Boston, PSG, 1983; pp 451–471.

4 Tizianello A, Deferrari G, Garibotto G, et al: Is amino acid imbalance harmful to patients in chronic renal failure? Kidney Int 1985;28:S79–S83.

5 Mitch WE, Walser M: Nutritional therapy of the uremic patients; in Brenner BM, Rector FC (eds): The Kidney. Philadelphia, Saunders, 1986, pp 1759–1790.

6 Tizianello A, Deferrari G, Garibotto G, et al: Abnormalities of amino acid and ketoacid metabolism in chronic renal failure; in Davison AM, 10th Congr Nephrology. Nephrology. London, Baillière, Tindall, 1988, vol II, pp 1011–1025.

7 Tizianello A, Deferrari G, Garibotto G, et al: Branched-chain amino acid metabolism in chronic renal failure. Kidney Int 1983;24:S17–S22.

8 Tizianello A, Deferrari G, Garibotto G, et al: Abnormalities in amino acid metabolism in patients with chronic renal failure. A pathophysiological approach to the nutritional treatment. I. Studies in the postabsorptive state. Contrib Nephrol 1987;55:1–10.

9 Deferrari G, Garibotto G, Robaudo C, et al: Leg metabolism of amino acids and ammonia in patients with chronic renal failure. Clin Sci 1985;69:143–151.

10 Deferrari G, Garibotto G, Robaudo C, et al: Glucose interorgan exchange in chronic renal failure. Kidney Int 1983;24:S115–S120.

11 De Fronzo RA, Smith D, Alvestrand A: Insulin action in uremia. Kidney Int 1983;24:S102–S114.

12 May RC, Hara Y, Kelly RA, et al: Branched-chain amino acid metabolism in rat muscle: abnormal regulation in acidosis. Am J Physiol 1987;252:E712–E718.

13 Tizianello A, Deferrari G, Garibotto G, et al: Renal metabolism of amino acids and ammonia in subjects with normal renal function and in patients with chronic renal insufficiency. J Clin Invest 1980;65:1162–1173.

14 Tizianello A, Deferrari G, Garibotto G, et al: Renal ammoniagenesis in the postprandial period. Contrib Nephrol 1985;47:44–57.

15 Tizianello A, Deferrari G, Garibotto G, et al: Amino acid metabolism and the liver in renal failure. Am J Clin Nutr 1980;33:1354–1362.

16 Deferrari G, Garibotto G, Robaudo C, et al: Splanchnic exchange of amino acids after amino acid ingestion in patients with chronic renal insufficiency. Am J Clin Nutr 1988;48:72–83.

17 Pardridge WM, Oldendorf WH: Transport of metabolic substrates through the blood-brain barrier. J Neurochem 1977;5:28–35.

18 Deferrari G, Garibotto G, Robaudo C, et al: Brain metabolism in uremia; in Kleinberger G, Ferenci P, Riederer P, Thaler H (eds): Advances in Hepatic Encephalopathy and Urea Cycle Diseases. Basel, Karger, 1984, pp 484–498.

19 Deferrari G, Garibotto G, Robaudo C, et al: Brain metabolism of amino acids and ammonia in patients with chronic renal insufficiency. Kidney Int 1981;20:505–510.

20 Tizianello A, Deferrari G, Garibotto G, et al: Influence of arterial branched-chain amino acid concentration on cerebral uptake of branched-chain amino acids and glycine in chronic renal insufficiency; in Walser M, Williamson JR (eds); Metabolism and Clinical Implications of Branched-Chain Amino and Ketoacids. New York, Elsevier/North-Holland, 1981, pp 581–586.

21 Wahren J, Felig P, Hagenfeldt L: Effect of protein ingestion on splanchnic and leg metabolism in normal man and in patients with diabetes mellitus. J Clin Invest 1976;57:979–999.

22 Deferrari G, Garibotto G, Robaudo C, et al: Abnormalities in blood profile of amino acids after a protein meal in patients with chronic renal failure: a premise for an imbalance in brain amino acid uptake. Kidney Int, in press.

23 Garibotto G, Deferrari G, Robaudo C, et al: Effect of protein meal on blood amino acid profile in patients with chronic renal failure. Metabolism, submitted.

24 Garibotto G, Deferrari G, Robaudo C, et al: Effect of amino acid ingestion on blood amino acid levels in patients with chronic renal failure. Am J Clin Nutr 1987;46:949–954.

25 Tizianello A, Deferrari G, Garibotto G, et al: Abnormal amino acid metabolism after amino acid ingestion in chronic renal failure. Kidney Int 1987;32:S181–185.

26 Harper AE, Benevenga NJ, Wohlhueter RM: Effects of ingestion of disproportionate amounts of amino acids. Physiol Rev 1970;50:428–458.

27 Morgan HE, Jefferson LS, Wolpert EB, et al: Regulation of protein synthesis in heart muscle. II. Effect of amino acid levels in insulin on ribosomal aggregation. J Biol Chem 1971;246:2152–2162.

28 Brenner BM, Meyer TW, Hostetter TH: Dietary protein intake and the progressive nature of kidney disease: the role of hemodynamically mediated glomerular sclerosis in aging, renal ablation, and intrinsic renal disease. N Engl J Med 1982;307:652–659.

Alberto Tizianello, MD, Istituto Scientifico di Medicina Interna, Section of Nephrology, Viale Benedetto XV, 6, I–16132 Genova (Italy)

Oldrizzi L, Maschio G, Rugiu C, et al. (eds): The Progressive Nature of Renal Disease: Myths and Facts. Contrib Nephrol. Basel, Karger, 1989, vol 75, pp 194–202

Nutritional and Metabolic Effects of Ten Years of Protein-Restricted Diet in Patients with Early Renal Failure

G. Toigo[a], *L. Oldrizzi*[b], *R. Situlin*[a], *G. Tamaro*[a], *L. Faccini*[a], *M. Russo*[a], *L. Campanacci*[a], *C. Rugiu*[b], *G. Maschio*[b], *G. F. Guarnieri*[a]

[a]University of Trieste, Institute of Medical Pathology, Trieste, and
[b]University of Verona, Division of Nephrology, Verona, Italy

A moderate and long-term restriction of protein and phosphorus intake has been advocated to retard the progression of renal failure in chronic glomerular diseases [1–4]. The requirements for nitrogen equilibrium in normal adults, allowing 30% for individual variation, are 0.6 g of high-quality proteins/kg of body weight/day [5]. It is not known whether the dietary nitrogen requirements in chronically uremic patients differ from those in normal subjects [6]. Experimental and clinical studies have shown that many abnormalities of protein metabolism are present in chronic uremia [3, 7, 8]. The pathogenesis of malnutrition in chronic uremia is probably multifactorial [8] and it is not known when these abnormalities of protein and energy metabolism appear during the progressive destruction of the kidneys. Therefore, it is not a priori known whether the long-term intake of 0.6–0.7 g of proteins/kg of body weight/day is adequate in patients with early renal insufficiency (ERF). If very low protein diets are to be regarded as safe, it is necessary to prove, by careful assessment of nutritional state, that their long-term use does not cause malnutrition. However, the nutritional adequacy of the protein-restricted diets used to slow the progression of renal diseases has been evaluated only in few studies, mostly performed after limited periods of treatment [8–10]. For these reasons we believe that, in order to avoid the risk of malnutrition, careful nutritional assessment is mandatory, to test if these low-protein diets are adequate to support normal nutritional status in treated patients.

In a previous study in 12 stable patients with ERF (average serum creatinine 2.1 mg/dl), treated for 52 months with a moderately low-protein diet, we reported that their nutritional state could be considered adequate [8]. Only very mild nutritional and metabolic abnormalities were present in some patients. We report here the results of nutritional state assessment in some of those patients after 5 further years of protein-restricted diet and, for comparison, the results of the first assessment in the same patients. The results of a previous nutritional study [7] on patients with advanced renal failure are reported as well.

For nutritional assessment, beside determining the anthropometric and biochemical indices, we also directly evaluated muscle protein metabolism, by measuring in needle biopsy specimens of skeletal muscle the concentration of noncollagen alkali-soluble proteins (ASP), of RNA and of DNA, and the activity of cathepsin D [7, 11–13]. As previously reported [12, 13], muscle DNA content in adults is considered a satisfactory reference standard, because in protein energy malnutrition the total number of nuclei in muscle is slightly affected. The ratio of muscle ASP, i.e. noncollagen proteins, to DNA is an index of a hypothetical muscle cell size [12, 13]. Total muscle RNA content, which is about 80% ribosomal RNA, and the RNA:DNA ratio are a measure of the capacity of the cell to synthesize proteins [12, 13]. According to many studies in animals and in humans, starvation and refeeding are accompanied by progressive changes in muscle RNA content, and in muscle protein synthesis and content [12, 13]. Muscle protein breakdown involves complex and poorly understood mechanisms, including several proteinases and inhibitors of their activity. Different proteolytic systems are active in skeletal muscle in different conditions [11, 14]. Cathepsin D is an acid lysosomal endopeptidase, whose activity changes in skeletal muscle in different metabolic and clinical conditions [11]. Many studies suggest that the lysosomal cathepsin D is involved in skeletal muscle proteolysis and is capable of degrading myofibrillar proteins [11]. Muscle proteinase activities determined in muscle extracts have been shown to follow rates of muscle protein degradation both in vivo and in vitro.

Patients and Methods

We previously examined 12 patients with ERF after 5 years of protein-restricted diet [8]: the nutritional status and muscle protein metabolism were assessed again in 8 (5 males) of the initial patients, after 5 further years of low-protein diets. Of the initial 12 patients, 3 were dialyzed and one was transferred to another center. The results of a previous nutritional study [7] in patients with advanced renal failure are reported for comparison.

Age, diagnosis, time on dietary treatment, dietary intake and routine blood chemistries of the patients are reported in table 1. No patient with systemic diseases or intercurrent illnesses was included in the study. No relevant changes of urinary protein excretion and systemic blood pressure were observed between the two assessments in the patients. Blood acid-base status and glucose tolerance were normal in all patients with ERF.

Methods for nutritional assessment and blood and muscle sampling and analysis were previously reported [7, 8, 11]. Statistical analysis was performed by means of SPSS/PC plus.

Table 1. Age, months on low-protein diet, principal laboratory data and dietary intake of the patients, expressed as mean ± SD

	ERF 1st assessment	p	ERF 2nd assessment	Advanced renal failure
Age, years	55 ± 7	–	60 ± 8	56 ± 13
Months on low-protein diet	52 ± 28	–	118 ± 11	–
Urea N, mg/dl	18 ± 11	n.s.	18 ± 8	84 ± 24
Creatinine, mg/dl	1.9 ± 0.8	n.s.	2.6 ± 1.7	10.0 ± 2.8
Glucose, mg/dl	105 ± 33	n.s.	94 ± 14	93 ± 15
Hemoglobin, g/dl	14.5 ± 1.6	0.029	13.2 ± 2.0	9.1 ± 1.9
Calcium, mg/dl	9.7 ± 0.4	n.s.	9.5 ± 0.5	7.8 ± 0.9
Phosphates, mg/dl	2.9 ± 0.3	n.s.	3.2 ± 0.7	5.3 ± 1.8
Valine/glycine	0.9 ± 0.3**	n.s.	1.1 ± 0.5	–
Phenylalanine/tyrosine	1.10 ± 0.14	n.s.	1.24 ± 0.15*	–
Essential AA/nonessential AA	0.44 ± 0.6*	n.s.	0.51 ± 0.09***	–
Dietary energy, kcal/kg DBW/day	29 ± 4	0.01	26 ± 3	33 ± 6
Dietary proteins, g/kg DBW/day	0.76 ± 0.13	n.s.	0.73 ± 0.09	0.77 ± 0.24

DBW = Desirable body weight; n.s. = not significant. Level of significance vs controls (Student's t-test): *$p < 0.001$; **$p < 0.01$; ***$p < 0.05$.
p values refer to statistical analysis (Student's *t*-test for paired data) between the first and second assessment in patients with ERF.
Diagnosis: GN, N:2; PN, N:2; PKD, N:1; VE, N:3.

Results

Dietary protein intakes in the patients with ERF were 0.76 ± 0.13 and 0.73 ± 0.09 g/kg desirable body weight/day, respectively, on the first and second assessment (table 1). Their energy intake was rather low: 29 ± 4 and 26 ± 3 kcal/kg/day.

The mean serum creatinine concentration of the 8 patients with ERF on protein-restricted diet increased, in more than 5 years, only from 1.9 ± 0.8 to 2.6 ± 1.7 mg/dl (table 1). In the meantime, blood hemoglobin levels significantly decreased and the ratios of serum amino acid levels remained slightly abnormal (our fasting normal values of the Val:Gly, Phe:Tyr and essential:nonessential amino acid ratios are 1.25 ± 0.47, 0.84 ± 0.13, 0.61 ± 0.09, respectively.

As to anthropometry, fat stores only slightly and not significantly decreased between the first and the second assessment (table 2).

Table 2. Anthropometric measurements of the patients, expressed as mean ± SD

	ERF 1st assessment	ERF 2nd assessment	Advanced renal failure
Body mass index	24.0 ± 1.4	23.0 ± 1.9	24 ± 4
Skinfold thickness			
Triceps (TST), mm	11.6 ± 6.5 (10)	9.0 ± 4.5 (12)	6.5 ± 4.2 (64)
Subscapular (SST), mm	11.9 ± 3.0 (10)	10.5 ± 2.9 (37)	8.4 ± 3.6 (64)
Arm muscle circumference (AMC), mm	244 ± 13 (10)	249 ± 8 (0)	216 ± 29 (36)
Arm muscle area (AMA), mm^2	4,750 ± 523 (10)	4,939 ± 334 (0)	3,654 ± 1,249 (36)

The percentages of values under the 5th percentiles are reported in parentheses.
Student's t-test for paired data did not show any significant difference between the first and the second assessment in the patients with ERF.

On the other hand, the serum content of protein synthesized in the visceral compartment significantly decreased in the patients with ERF after 5 further years of low-protein diet (table 3).

As reported in table 4, muscle DNA concentration and the RNA:DNA and ASP:DNA ratios did not significantly change between the first and the second assessment. Only muscle fat content was significantly lower than in controls on the second assessment in the patients with ERF. Cathepsin D activity was significantly decreased on the second assessment in patients with ERF, whereas it was normal in patients with advanced renal failure.

Many significant correlations (table 5) were found also on the second assessment among the nutritional indices and plasma essential amino acids and some muscular indices.

In patients with advanced renal failure, on the contrary, anthropometric measurements were often abnormal, and serum protein content, especially albumin and complement fractions, were below normal ranges in a large percentage of patients (tables 2, 3). The increased concentration of muscle DNA in patients with advanced renal failure was an index of reduced muscle mass. Both RNA:DNA and ASP:DNA ratios were lower than in controls in these patients (table 4).

Table 3. Serum protein content, expressed as mean ± SD

	Lower normal values	ERF 1st assessment	p	ERF 2nd assessment	Advanced renal failure
Total proteins, g/dl	6.3	7.3 ± 0.5 (0)	n.s.	7.1 ± 1.1 (0)	6.8 ± 0.9 (24)
Albumin, mg/dl	3,500	4,593 ± 521 (0)	0.002	3,340 ± 413 (71)	2,893 ± 593 (87)
Transferrin, mg/dl	205	243 ± 72 (14)	0.016	145 ± 36 (100)	247 ± 78 (40)
Pseudocholinesterase, U/l	1,900	2,191 ± 817 (14)	n.s.	2,637 ± 753 (13)	2,055 ± 674 (33)
C3, mg/dl	55	75 ± 12 (0)	0.001	46 ± 8 (86)	—
	100	—	—	—	95 ± 39 (62)
C3 activator, mg/dl	10	14 ± 3 (0)	0.022	11 ± 2 (14)	
	18	—	—	—	19 ± 5 (54)

The percentages of values under the normal ranges are reported in parentheses. n.s. = Not significant.
p values refer to statistical analysis (Student's t-test for paired data) between the first and the second assessment in patients with ERF.

Table 4. Muscle DNA, RNA, ASP, water and fat content, and cathepsin D activity (CDA), in muscle biopsy specimens, expressed as mean ± SD

	Controls (n = 20)	ERF 1st assessment	ERF 2nd assessment	Advanced renal failure
DNA, mg/100 g wet wt	34 ± 8	39 ± 4	37 ± 10	47 ± 17**
RNA, mg/100 g wet wt	77 ± 22	83 ± 7	71 ± 7	71 ± 25
ASP, g/100 g wet wt	18 ± 2	19 ± 3	17 ± 3	16.4 ± 2.8
RNA/DNA, mg/mg	2.3 ± 0.6	2.0 ± 0.5	2.0 ± 0.5	1.65 ± 0.75**
ASP/DNA, mg/mg	554 ± 106	472 ± 41	499 ± 138	388 ± 127**
Water, g/100 g of FFS	306 ± 58	309 ± 37	307 ± 29	340 ± 46
Fats, g/100 g of FFS	25 ± 17	21 ± 15	11 ± 7*	18 ± 12
CDA, mU/100 mg wet wt	94 ± 12	80 ± 14	68 ± 19*	83 ± 25
CDA/DNA, mU/μg	3.0 ± 0.7	2.2 ± 0.3	1.9 ± 0.8*	2.39 ± 0.99

FFS = Fat-free solids; ASP = alkali-soluble proteins. Level of significance vs controls (Student's t-test): *$p < 0.025$; **$p < 0.005$. CDA was determined in 9 controls.
Student's t-test for paired data did not show any significant difference between the first and the second assessment in the patients with ERF.

Table 5. Significant correlations ($p < 0.05$ or lower) in patients with ERF (second assessment)

Creatinine	Dietary proteins (% of total energy)	−0.78
	Plasma valine	−0.69
	Plasma leucine	−0.71
	Plasma lysine	−0.86
	Plasma phenylalanine	−0.76
	Plasma methionine	0.79
Energy/kg DBW	Cath D:ASP	−0.81
	Plasma valine	−0.85
	Plasma leucine	−0.88
Dietary proteins, % of total energy	Plasma valine	0.91
	Plasma isoleucine	0.84
	Plasma leucine	0.91
Dietary proteins, g/kg DBW	Cath D:DNA	−0.73
Carbohydrates/kg DBW	Plasma valine	−0.78
	Plasma leucine	−0.83
	Plasma lysine	−0.76
	Plasma tyrosine	−0.76
	Plasma phenylalanine	−0.77
Energy intake	Muscle ASP	0.74
Dietary fats, % of total energy	% DBW	0.69
Cath B	AMA	0.72
RNA:DNA	ASP:DNA	0.84
TST	SST	0.72
Plasma valine	Plasma isoleucine	0.92
	Plasma leucine	0.98
Plasma isoleucine	Plasma leucine	0.92
Plasma tyrosine	Plasma phenylalanine	0.96

Discussion and Conclusions

Results obtained in the present study by anthropometric measurements, biochemical determinations and direct skeletal muscle analysis show that the nutritional state of the patients with ERF on long-term low-protein diet tended to slowly worsen between the 5th and the 10th year of diet.

More severe nutritional abnormalities were present in patients with advanced renal failure.

The diet prescribed to the patients was 0.6 g of protein and 40 kcal of energy/kg desirable body weight/day [8], but their actual energy intake was lower than prescribed, especially on the second assessment. Anthropometric indices were only moderately decreased in patients with ERF and stable between the two assessments. On the contrary, patients with advanced renal failure showed a frequent decrease of fat and muscle stores, that were often below the 5th percentiles of a normal population. The serum levels of proteins synthesized by the liver were strongly decreased in the patients with ERF on the second assessment, and this suggests that dietary intake was inadequate to maintain their visceral protein synthesis. Serum protein levels were often low in patients with advanced renal failure. Muscle protein synthesis and content, evaluated, respectively, by the RNA:DNA and ASP:DNA ratios, were normal in patients with ERF on both assessments. Muscle protein synthetic capacity and content were significantly decreased in patients with advanced renal failure. Muscle protein degradation rate, evaluated by the measurement of cathepsin D activity, was definitely decreased in patients with ERF on the second assessment. We previously reported a very low cathepsin D activity also in malnourished patients on maintenance hemodialysis and in other groups of chronically malnourished nonuremic patients [11, 12]. These findings suggest that in the skeletal muscle of patients with ERF, after about 10 years of low-protein diet, protein degradation – but not protein synthesis and content – is low. In these patients the low cathepsin D activity may represent an adaptive mechanism of protein sparing during long-term low-protein diets [15]. Contrary to results obtained in uremic rats, in which an increased muscle protein breakdown has been reported [16, 17], a lower protein flux, i.e. a lower rate of both protein synthesis and breakdown, were observed in our chronically uremic patients, in agreement with other studies in humans [18–21]. In these patients the unbalance between the normal catabolism and the reduced synthesis of muscle proteins is probably relevant to the low muscle protein content (low ASP:DNA ratio).

The significant direct correlations between the dietary intake of proteins and the serum concentrations of branched chain amino acids suggest a persistent effect of dietary protein intake on branched chain amino acid metabolism. Muscle protein content and cathepsin D activity were also correlated to energy and protein intake, as previously reported in other groups of patients.

It has been suggested that the causes of malnutrition in uremia are more complex than simply impaired nutritional intake and are also related to uremic toxins and metabolic abnormalities [22, 23]. However, it is likely that the main cause of the nutritional abnormalities, observed on the second assessment in our patients with ERF, is the reduced dietary intake, because their mean serum creatinine level was only 2.6 mg/dl. Further long-term studies are needed to evaluate if a more adequate dietary intake is equally effective in slowing the progression of renal diseases and can maintain a better nutritional state. However, it may be difficult to maintain for many years these patients on a reduced protein intake and, simultaneously, on an optimal energy intake.

In conclusion, this study suggests that dietary intake was not adequate to maintain normal muscle and visceral protein metabolism in patients with ERF after 10 years of protein-restricted diet. These abnormalities may be primarily related to the low energy intake of both groups of patients. However, considering both the risks and the benefits of these diets, it should be pointed out that renal function remained practically stable for about 10 years at least in 8 of the initial 12 patients. Anyway, our results suggest that a careful monitoring of nutritional and metabolic state is advisable in patients with ERF on long-term protein-restricted diets. These patients should be encouraged to increase their energy intake and probably in some cases, they should receive energy supplements [24].

References

1 Maschio G, Oldrizzi L, Tessitore N, et al: Effects of dietary protein and phosphoru restriction on the progression of early renal failure. Kidney Int 1982;22:371–376.

2 Strauch M, Giovannetti S (eds): Low protein diet and progression of chronic rena failure. Contrib Nephrol 1986;53.

3 Kopple JD, Winchester J, Massry SG, et al: An update on nutrition and metabolism ii kidney disease. Kidney Int 1987;32(suppl 22).

4 Mitch WE: Nutritional therapy and the progression of renal insufficiency; in Mitch WE Klahr S (eds): Nutrition and the Kidney. Boston, Little, Brown, 1988; pp 154–179.

5 Kopple JD, Swenseid ME: Amino acid and keto acid diet for therapy in renal failure Nephron 1977;18:1–2.

6 Hirschberg RR, Kopple JD: Requirements for protein, calories and fat in the predialysi patient; in Mitch WE, Klahr S (eds): Nutrition and the Kidney. Boston, Little, Brown 1988, pp 131–153.

7 Guarnieri G, Toigo G, Situlin R, et al: Muscle biopsy studies in chronically uremi patients: evidence for malnutrition. Kidney Int 1983;24(suppl 16):S187–S193.

8 Guarnieri G, Toigo G, Situlin R, et al: Nutritional assessment in patients with earl renal insufficiency on long-term low protein diet. Contrib Nephrol 1986;53:40–50.

9 Lucas PA, Meadows JH, Roberts DE, et al: The risks and benefits of a low protein essential amino acid-keto acid diet. Kidney Int 1986;29:995–1003.

10 Acchiardo SR, Moore LW, Cockrell S: Does low protein diet halt the progression c renal insufficiency? Clin Nephrol 1986;25:289–294.

11 Guarnieri G, Toigo G, Situlin R, et al: Muscle cathepsin D activity and RNA, DNA an protein content in maintenance hemodialysis patients; in Horl WF, Heidland A (eds):

Proteases: Potential Role In Health and Disease. New York, Plenum Press, 1984, pp 533–543.

12 Guarnieri G, Toigo G, Situlin R, et al: Direct biochemical analysis of human muscle tissue in hospital malnutrition. J Parent Ent Nutr 1987;11:55S–63S.

13 Guarnieri G, Toigo G, Situlin R: Proteinase activity as well as DNA, RNA and protein content in human skeletal muscle in malnutrition and in disease states; in Dietz G, Peter K, Steibereithner K, Wolfram G, Hauser B (eds): Wertigkeit metabolischer Parameter in der parenteralen Ernährung. Klinische Ernährung, 1987, vol 29, pp 3–12.

14 Jahoor F, Wolfe RR: Regulation of protein catabolism. Kidney Int 1987;32(suppl 22):S81–S93.

15 Waterlow JC, Garlick PJ, Millward DJ: The effects of nutrition and hormones on protein turnover in muscle; in Protein Turnover in Mammalian Tissues and in Whole Body. Amsterdam, Biomedical Press, 1978, pp 625–695.

16 Harter HR, Karl IE, Klahr S, et al: Effects of reduced renal mass and dietary protein intake on amino acid release and glucose uptake by rat muscle in vitro. J Clin Invest 1979;64:513–523.

17 Mitch WE, Clark AS: Muscle protein turnover in uremia. Kidney Int 1983;24(suppl 16):S2–S8.

18 Conley SB, Rose GM, Robson AM, et al: Effects of dietary intake and hemodialysis on protein turnover in uremic children. Kidney Int 1980;17:837–846.

19 Defronzo RA, Smith D, Alvestrand A: Insulin action in uremia. Kidney Int 1983;24(suppl 16):S102–S114.

20 Alvestrand A: Amino acid metabolism in patients with chronic renal failure. Clin Nutr 1985;4(suppl):14.

21 Deferrari G, Garibotto G, Robaudo C, et al: Leg metabolism of amino acids and ammonia in patients with chronic renal failure. Clin Sci 1985;69:143–151.

22 Feinstein EI, Kopple JD: Severe wasting and malnutrition in a patient undergoing maintenance dialysis. Am J Nephrol 1985;5:398–405.

23 Wassner SJ, Bergstrom J, Brusilow SW, et al: Protein metabolism in renal failure: abnormalities and possible mechanisms. Am J Kidney Dis 1986;7:285–291.

24 Gretz N, Lasserre J, Strauch M: Caloric supplements for patients on low-protein diets? Nephron 1988;50:129–132.

G. F. Guarnieri, MD, University of Trieste, Istituto di Patologia Medica, Ospedale di Cattinara, I–34149 Trieste (Italy)

Oldrizzi L, Maschio G, Rugiu C, et al. (eds): The Progressive Nature of Renal Disease: Myths and Facts. Contrib Nephrol. Basel, Karger, 1989, vol 75, pp 203–208

The Optimal Protein Intake in Patients with Early Chronic Renal Failure

Lamberto Oldrizzi, Carlo Rugiu, Giuseppe Maschio
Division of Nephrology, University Hospital, Verona, Italy

The optimal protein intake for patients with reduced renal function who are not undergoing regular dialysis treatment must satisfy these aims: (a) to be well accepted by patient; (b) to preserve a normal nutritional status; (c) to prevent the glomerular hypertension; (d) to slow the progression of renal failure towards uremia and dialysis.

Nowadays two types of diets are commonly used in these patients. The first one is very low in protein, providing about 15–20 g of protein per day with a supplementation of essential amino acids [1]. The second is a moderately low-protein diet that supplies 0.55–0.60 g/kg body weight (0.35 g of high biologic value) without any supplementation and/or artificial food. In our experience this latter diet can satisfy the above-cited conditions for an optimal protein intake.

We tried to support our assumption on the basis of two different research guidelines: (a) What are the effects on renal function of an oral protein load when given to patients kept on a diet providing 0.6 g/kg of protein? (b) Is there any difference in renal function when the patient is eating the low-protein or a normal-protein diet?

Oral Protein Loads

First of all, we analyze the problem concerning the oral protein loads and we state the concept of renal functional reserve. In healthy subjects an oral protein load increases both the renal plasma flow and the glomerular filtration rate (GFR) [2, 3]. These changes are somewhat related to each other. Thus, the increase in GFR can be considered as the effect of increased glomerular flows and pressures. The difference between resting and stimulated GFR has been defined as renal functional reserve [4]. In healthy subjects the absence of renal reserve may be the equivalent of hyperfiltration, since failing any increase in GFR should mean that the available nephrons are working at their maximum level [4].

Although a reduction in renal functional mass reduces the magnitude of renal reserve, we can assume, when a patient maintains some renal reserve, that glomerular flows are not maximal and thus no hyperfiltration is present.

The oral protein load protocol we used can be briefly summarized as follows. GFR, as iothalamate clearance [5], was assessed 90 min before and 120 min after the protein load, consisting of 1.5 g of protein per kilogram in the form of grilled red meat, ingested within 30 min. The scheme should guarantee a true evaluation of changes in renal function, the peak time of stimulated GFR being between 120 and 150 min after the protein load [6].

The results obtained in patients treated with a diet containing 0.6 g of protein show a persisting renal reserve. This fact has been shown in different situations of reduced renal mass: i.e. in patients with solitary kidneys and slightly reduced renal function [7, 8]. These patients, kept on a long-term dietary protein restriction, when tested with our standard oral protein load, experienced an increase in GFR (renal reserve) of 48.7 ± 16.7 ml/min (from 59 to 10.7 ml/min) not different from that recorded in a control population. The preservation of renal reserve was also evident in patients with more advanced functional derangement [9]. Despite a supposed lower number of surviving nephrons, GFR rose, after the protein load, from 22.5 ± 10.6 to 60.1 ± 32.8 ml/min (t: 3.44; p: 0.006), corresponding to a renal reserve of 37.6 ± 23.8 ml/min. Thus, it seemed evident that patients with reduced functional renal mass maintained effective renal reserve when kept on moderate dietary protein restriction.

Taken together, the results of these studies support the idea that patients with renal failure and treated with a 0.6 protein diet fail to show glomerular hypertension in their kidneys. Unfortunately, some problems might decrease the clinical validity of these results: the short time of observation; the high protein amount ingested during the test, far from that a subject can introduce with an usual meal; the unknown rate of individual intestinal absorption of protein we gave.

Short-Term Comparative Studies

A first effort to overcome these problems has been represented by a short-term study (over 3 days) comparing the effects on renal function of a normal and a low-protein diet. We studied 10 patients with various degrees of renal damage, all kept on long-term dietary protein restriction. Their basal GFR ranged from 20 to 45 ml/min (mean 27 ± 14) [10]. On day 1 and

3 the patients were kept on diet P1, on day 2 on diet P2. Diet P1 provided 0.6 g of protein and 600 mg of phosphate, whereas diet P2 1.0 g/kg of protein and 1,300 mg of phosphate. The diets were isocaloric. The radioisotopic assessment of changes in GFR from day 1 (mean 27 ± 14 ml/min) to day 2 (mean 39 ± 21), and from day 2 to day 3 (mean 31 ± 18 ml/min), showed that a slight increase in protein intake was able to raise GFR.

Moreover, the renal reserve, that is the increment in GFR on day 2, was inversely related to basal protein intake, available from nitrogen balance (recorded before the study) ($r = -0.75$; $p = 0.005$). A similar relationship was evident also between renal reserve and phosphaturia and thus, indirectly, with phosphate intake ($r = -0.79$; $p = 0.001$). Actually, these results gave further support to a protective role of 0.6 protein diet in renal failure.

Long-Term Comparative Studies

The long-term evaluation of the different effects on renal function between normal or high-protein and low-protein diets has been carried out with randomized or self-controlled studies. As far as the normal subjects are concerned, a very interesting observation was made by Wiseman et al. [11], i.e. that renal function is influenced by the dietary protein contents. In this study GFR was recorded in 18 vegans, 16 lactovegetarians and 18 omnivores subjects.

The results were obtained before and after a 6-month follow-up on different diets: the omnivores ate 1.3 g/kg of protein (70% animal), the vegans 0.95 g/kg and the lactovegetarians 1.03 g/kg (35% animal). Mean GFR was significantly lower in vegans (100 ± 13 ml/min/1.73 m^2) than in the omnivores (113 ± 16 ml/min/1.73 m^2), whereas lactovegetarians had intermediate values (105 ± 16 ml/min/1.73 m^2). Moreover, as microalbuminuria as diastolic blood pressure values were significantly higher in the omnivore group. The randomized studies satisfy the statistic rules for comparative evaluations in clinical trials [12]. Besides the study presented by Dr. Locatelli elsewhere in this book, I would like to remind the reader of the Groningen study on the effects of low-protein diet [13]. The comparison of long-term effects on progression of renal failure of both 0.6 and 0.4 g/kg protein diets with those of free diets was made in 228 patients. Both the average rate of decrease in reciprocal creatinine and the renal survival analysis showed that a moderate dietary protein restriction had a protective role on kidneys function.

Although controlled study design is believed to be less accurate, the self-controlled design, in which each patient serves as his own control, can produce results that are statistically valid with far fewer patients than would otherwise be required [14]. We present the results of two of such studies. The first one is by Schaap et al. [15]. They assessed in a group of patients with early renal failure, the changes in GFR and renal plasma flow after 2 months of follow-up. During the first month, the patients had a low-protein intake (40 g/day); in the second study period, they were kept on a normal protein diet, providing 80 g/day. The results showed that a switch from a low-protein to a normal-protein intake caused an increase in GFR (from 48 to 58 ml/min/1.73 m^2) and renal plasma flow (ERPF) (from 205 to 243 ml/min/1.73 m^2). At the same time, urinary protein excretion rose significantly during the high protein period (1.6 vs 1.0 g/24 h). The authors concluded that prolonged high protein intake is followed by changes in renal function bearing glomerular hypertension.

The second study is a clinical experience from Verona Group. By using the self-controlled design, we evaluate in a small group of patients ($n = 7$) with moderate renal failure the effects of a low (40 g/day) and slightly reduced (60 g/day) protein intakes.

Each patient had been studied during 3 periods: (period A) diet providing 40 g, averaged 12 months; (period B) diet providing 60 g, lasted 9 months; (period C) diet providing 40 g, averaged 9 months. To avoid any carry-over effects due to the different content in creatine and creatinine, a washout period between period A and B and period B and C was planned.

No changes in blood pressure and drug therapy were made during the study. The computation of patients' dietary intakes at home showed that the protein intakes averaged 41.1 g/day in period A, 57.1 g/day in period B, and 41.3 g/day in period C.

GFR, as iothalamate clearance, seemed to be closely related to the dietary protein content. It changed from 43 to 46 ml/min in period A; at the start of period B, it was 52 ml/min but it decreased to 40 ml/min at the end of this period. In period C GFR showed a new stabilization, changing from 40 to 45 ml/min. The average value of proteinuria was higher in period B (1.3 g/day) when compared with the values observed in periods A (0.55) and C (0.8). Although this parameter is not a specific index of renal functional deterioration it is known to reflect to some extent glomerular hypertension [16] and to be related with a worst prognosis in chronic renal failure [17].

The results of this study suggest that when dietary protein intake exceeds 0.6 g/kg, functional changes in surviving nephrons happen. Actually, a new aspect is represented by data collected in period C; they apparently suggest that changes in renal function observed in period B are to some degree reversible. So far we do not know how long an increased protein intake has to last to produce organic and thus not reversible damage. Our data indicate that even after 9 months restoring an adequate protein diet could stabilize renal hemodynamics.

Conclusions

Finally, as far as the patients' compliance with the diet is concerned, we recently assessed it in a population of 390 patients, followed for a mean period of 4.5 years. When done by means of well-known methods (urea nitrogen appearance, phosphaturia/24 h, dietary recalls), the compliance was found to be satisfactory (estimated protein intake within 0.5 and 0.7 g/kg of body weight) in 77% of patients [17].

In conclusion, these suggestions come from clinical studies on the effects of a diet providing 0.6 g/kg of protein: (a) a good patients compliance; (b) no nutritional adverse effects [18]; (c) prevention of glomerula hypertension; (d) reduction of rate of progression of functional deterioration [13, 17–19].

References

1 Hirschberg R, Kopple JD: Requirements for protein, calories, and fat in the predialysis patient; in Mitch WE, Klahr S (eds): Nutrition and the Kidney. Boston, Little Brown, 1988, pp 131–153.

2 Mizuira S, Hayashi I, Ozawa T, Hirata K, Takano M, Sasaki Y: Effects of an oral protein load on glomerular filtration rate in healthy controls and nephrotic patients. Nephron 1988;48:101–106.

3 Rodriguez-Iturbe B, Herrera J, Garcia R: Relationship between glomerular filtration rate and renal blood flow at different levels of protein-induced hyperfiltration in man. Clin Sci 1988;47:11–15.

4 Bosch JP, Lew S, Glabman S, Lauer A: Renal hemodynamic changes in humans. Response to protein loading in normal and diseased kidneys. Am J Med 1986;81:809–815.

5 Ott NT, Wilson DN: A simple technique for estimating GFR with subcutaneous injection of ^{125}I iothalamate. Mayo Clin Proc 1975;50:664–668.

6 Laville M, Hadj-Aissa A, Pozet N, Le Bras JH, Labeeuw M, Zech P: Restrictions on use of creatinine clearance for measurements of renal functional reserve. Proc 5th Int Congr on Nutrition and Metabolsm in Renal Disease, Strasbourg, 1988, A103.

7 Rugiu C, Oldrizzi L, Maschio G: Effects of an oral protein load on GFR in patients with solitary kidneys. Kidney Int 1986;32(suppl 22):S29–S31.

8 Rugiu C, Oldrizzi L, Gammaro L, Tonon M, Maschio G: Glomerular filtration rate variations in patients with solitary kidneys after a protein load. Uremia Inv 1986;9:159–163.

9 Oldrizzi L, Rugiu C, Maschio G: Effects of an oral protein load in patients with chronic renal failure before and after angiotensin II blockade. Nephron, 1989;52:174–177.

10 Oldrizzi L, Rugiu C, Maschio G: Effects of different protein intakes on renal function and nitrogen metabolism in patients with early renal failure. Proc 4th Int Congr on Nutrition and Metabolism in Renal Disease, Williamsburg, 1985, A65.
11 Wiseman MJ, Hunt R, Goodwin A, Gross JL, Keen H, Viberti GC: Dietary composition and renal function in healthy subjects. Nephron 1987;46:37–42.
12 Spodick DH: The randomized controlled clinical trials. Scientific and ethical bases. Am J Med 1982;73:420–425.
13 Rosman JB, Ter Wee PM, Meijer S, Piers-Becht T, Sluiter WJ, Donker AJM: Prospective randomised trial of early dietary protein restriction in chronic renal failure. Lancet 1984;ii:1291–1295.
14 Louis TA, Lavori PW, Bailar JC II, Polansky M: Crossover and self controlled study in clinical research. N Engl J Med 1984;310:24–29.
15 Schaap GH, Bilo HJG, Alferink THR, Oe PL, Donker AJM: The effect of a high protein intake on renal function of patients with chronic renal insufficiency. Nephron 1987;47:1–6.
16 Brenner BM, Meyer TW, Hostetter TH: The role of hemodynamically mediated glomerular injury in the pathogenesis of progressive glomerular sclerosis in aging, renal ablation, and intrinsic renal disease. N Engl J Med 1982;308:652–659.
17 Oldrizzi L, Rugiu C, Maschio G: The Verona experience with the use of low protein diets. Kidney Int, in press.
18 Guarnieri GF, Toigo G, Situlin R, et al: Nutritional assessment in patients with early renal insufficiency of long-term low-protein diet. Contrib Nephrol 1986;53:40–50.
19 Maschio G, Oldrizzi L, Rugiu C: The effects of dietary protein restriction on the course of early renal failure; in Brenner BM, Stein JH (eds): The Progressive Nature of Renal Disease. New York, Churchill & Livingstone, 1986, p 203.

Lamberto Oldrizzi, MD, Divisione di Nefrologia, Ospedale Civile Maggiore, I–37126 Verona (Italy)

Subject Index